T0121680

SOCIAL WORK
IN THE
HOSPITAL SETTING

INTERVENTIONS

César M. Garcés Carranza, DSW

Summer 2012

Order this book online at www.trafford.com
or email orders@trafford.com

Most Trafford titles are also available at major online book retailers.

© Copyright 2013 César M. Garcés Carranza, DSW.
All rights reserved. No part of this publication may be reproduced, stored in a retrieval
system, or transmitted, in any form or by any means, electronic, mechanical, photocopying,
recording, or otherwise, without the written prior permission of the author.

Printed in the United States of America.

ISBN: 978-1-4669-9309-9 (sc)
ISBN: 978-1-4669-9310-5 (e)

Trafford rev. 06/18/2013

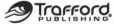 www.trafford.com

North America & international
toll-free: 1 888 232 4444 (USA & Canada)
phone: 250 383 6864 ♦ fax: 812 355 4082

DEDICATION

This Book is dedicated to
my parents Luis and Domitila
and to my sister Cristina

TABLE OF CONTENTS

ACKNOWLEDGEMENTS

IT IS ALWAYS A good idea for all of us to pay tribute to the people who have helped us with our projects in this life. I am not an exception when it comes to this good idea, for so many people have helped to mold and shape my ideas about social work in a hospital setting. First, I was lucky enough to land a job in the Bronx Lebanon Hospital in the South Bronx twenty three years ago. It is in this hospital that I have been brought to life about the historical link between social workers and the hospital. Moreover, since this is a busy hospital that deals with every possible medical as well as every psycho-social issue in the world, I have been left alone to figure it all out by myself. I want to thank the hospital administrators and doctors and nurses for being busy, overwhelmed even, because their dedication to their patients has made it possible to be something of a pioneer in the field of social work. I have not had a manual or a guidebook, but still I have been a social worker in the Emergency Room, the Intensive Care Unit and the Medical/Surgical Units of this hospital for almost a quarter of a century. I have had the maximum amount of time in this hospital to figure out exactly what social workers should be doing in hospitals in the first place. In addition to hospital staff, and social work colleagues; Sherri Stewart, Luz Rendon, Wendy Peguero, Pauline Linton, and Luz Holguin; I also wish to acknowledge Yeshiva University (WWSSW), along with Professors,

Dr. Louis Levitt, Dr. Norman Linzer, and Dr. Susan Mason. These people built a mind inside of me, and for that I will always be grateful. There are more people to thank; they are Dr. Nilda Valentin, Dr. Nicholas Dávila and Aracelia Jimenez for their friendship and support throughout the years. There is the Neuropsychiatric Institute staff to thank, where I have a private practice for the past twenty three years. There are so many fine psychotherapists at the Institute; they have sterling minds and I just wish to acknowledge their help throughout the years. Last, I want to thank my dearest wife Ellen for putting up with all the time spent away from home. Without her emotional support, and her good common sense I truly would have failed to publish this book. Also, I do not want to forget my good children Nicholas and Rachel, and my brothers and sister for their support has been invaluable. I love their way they look at life; they are so healthy and mature. I am proud of their lives and their choices in this life. At the very end, I would like to thank my patients, for they are the ones who have grown me up and cured me. They have curiously enough shown me the road less traveled, for without my patients I would not know the things I know. Thank you all for your contributions to this book on Social Work in the Hospital Setting-Interventions.

INTRODUCTION

M Y OBJECTIVE IN THE following work is to describe the different interventions used by social workers who work with the families of patients admitted to hospital: to the Emergency Room (ER), Intensive Care Unit (ICU), and General Medical Units. With all of the interventions explained, however, I continually place the emphasis on the communication that takes place between the medical personnel (doctors/nurses), and the families of patients. The kind of social worker I am ensures that the emotional needs of both patients and patients' families are met, which means that along with psychotherapy and counseling, I solve psychosocial problems as well.

I am a social worker in the Bronx Lebanon Hospital Center. The hospital is located in the South Bronx, which is one of the poorest neighborhoods in the United States. Even though the people who live near and around the hospital are poor, still the neighborhood turns out to be home to an extremely diverse group of people. The streets are filled with immigrants from almost all over the world. Once again, what is different about this diverse population is the fact that almost fifty per cent (50%) of the population lives below the poverty level. In addition, the citizens from the South Bronx live with chronic illness, such as AIDS, asthma, and diabetes. Moreover, the psychosocial problems are rife: gang activity, drug abuse, prostitution, homelessness, child abuse, elder abuse, and domestic violence are but a few of the common problems faced by people who live in the South Bronx (Bronx Lebanon Hospital, 2007).

One of my intentions in this book is to discover myself in the history (and traditions) of social work, to understand once and for all that the work I do at Bronx Lebanon Hospital has been done before by other social workers before me. Thus, in this book I do something very important: I trace the entrance of the social worker into the hospital setting, but especially into the ER, and later into the ICU, and eventually into the Medical Surgical Units. For instance, I write about Dr. Richard Cabot from the Massachusetts General Hospital, who in 1905 was the first doctor to invite social workers into the hospital to make certain social work interventions that heretofore had not been made.

This book on Social Work Interventions in the Hospital Setting is not really a history of social work, however, for I do not remain stuck in the past. I write about now, and what I do as a social worker today in the Bronx Lebanon Hospital in the South Bronx. Generally, my patients are very sick; they are often at risk of dying. The families suffer twice sometimes, because the medical staff does not communicate well with them. This means that from the time their loved one enters the hospital, they are in the dark. Everything about the condition of the patient is somehow unknown. Every question goes unanswered. This is where I enter the picture. I explain the situation in human terms, which make sense to family members. I guide the families through a vast labyrinth (medical bureaucracy), which can often seem cruel. Ultimately, I arrange for the patient to be discharged from the hospital, but at the same time I prepare families for realities about a loved one. It might be the case that family members are facing the patient's true condition for the very first time. This means that the families were in denial about something like drug addiction to prescription pills or in denial about the patient's insistence on having unprotected sex, taking the chance of transmitting Hepatitis C to significant others.

My experience as a social worker in the ER, ICU, and General Medical Unit is extensive. I am proud of the different roles I have played at Bronx Lebanon Hospital. I have been that crucial mediator needed between doctor and patient. Over the last twenty three years, I have helped many patients and their families to recover. For example, in the Intensive Care Unit (ICU) I have been and am often to this day the go-between, [between doctor and patient] who accompanies the family members during the admission of their loved one. I help families work through the terrible stress and anxiety associated with having a loved one in the ER or the ICU. I am often dealing with explosive emotions. Family members are like time bombs ready to go off. I am able to intervene and bring sense and sanity to a very volatile situation. Just like the doctor or the nurse never abandons the patient, so I too [the social worker] never abandon the patient, except the social worker never abandons the families as well. I do not just intervene; I educate the family. I use sense and sensibility and understanding. These are major tools. Once again, I am very proud to be a part of an expert professional team currently located in the Bronx Lebanon Hospital Center in the South Bronx, New York.

I wrote this book because I believe it is important for social workers to teach the medical staff (doctors/nurses), administrators and the public about the importance of their interventions with patients, families, and all other systems.

I believe that the value of knowing about these interventions will help to make social workers more an integral part of every health care organization, but especially a vital part of hospitals.

It is my strong opinion that social workers belong in the ER, as well as the ICU, and in any and every unit of General Medicine. Social workers provide Clinical Services, as well as a myriad number of Concrete Services. Social workers help patients and their families to overcome the crisis at hand, such as even the admission to the hospital, or sudden death of a loved one, or an instance of domestic violence, child abuse, elder abuse, homelessness, drug abuse, or chronic alcohol abuse. Furthermore, the social worker is the ideal discharge planner, as he/she knows the entire case history of the patient like no other member of the medical team.

Social work is a unique profession that has had to change directions on a number of occasions. Its history is sui generis (unique—one of a kind). Social work as a profession has made adjustments, but it has always come back again ever more adaptable. In this case, of social workers and the essential work they do in hospitals, I hope that this book serves as guide to social workers and other health care professionals, in their daily interventions with patients and families. I want my effort there to contribute to overall efforts of social workers; to alleviate suffering and give both patients and families the tools needed in order to return their lives to homeostasis, to balance, to regained health, and a sense of new found confidence in those people they have learned to call "helper."

Author
César M. Garcés, Carranza, PhD
September 2012

CHAPTER ONE

Chronological History of Social Work in the United States

This summary represents a chronological recompilation of the origin of Social Work in the United States.

S OCIAL WORK, AS A profession has its origin in the 19th century. It starts as a movement that concerns the poor. The movement for the poor started principally in England and the United States. Up until this time, poor people in history were not in any way noticed or singled out for special regard, by monarchies or by the nobility or the merchant classes. Even after the end of Feudalism, poor people were viewed as a direct threat to the social order. However, as the monarchies of Europe gave way to more democratic forms of government, especially in England, and as the concept of a civil society was extended, people could not help but acknowledge the poor. The poor suddenly seemed to be everywhere, but especially the poor chimney sweep children were noticed on the streets of London, Dublin and Edinburgh. While they had always been there, for the first time, now, they were seen. Their plight was recognized.

By 1850, even Tory government (conservatives) in England took note of the poor, and began to create and organize a help system that would specifically minister to the poor. In England, something called the Poor Law helped to classify the poor into different categories: the able poor, the handicaps, and the lazy ones. This system was one of the first typologies in Europe that recognized that not all the poor could be thrown into one big pile.

What helped to hasten the government's aid of the poor in the beginning of the 19th century was the Industrial Revolution. At this time, the great advances in technological and scientific knowledge ended up being the precipitating factor that caused the large migrations of people to the new urban areas. Cities were transformed into different kinds of spaces. However, with more people ending up in cities, this introduced many new social problems that had not existed before all the wonderful new gadgets that made life so much easier. With so many people concentrated in smaller spaces, the social movements that catered to the poor expanded. (Barker, R. L.,1998).

Running alongside the government's efforts to aid the poor, were the missionary movements that grew out of Protestant theology. Some of the efforts of these missions (Urban missions) tried to solve the problems that were becoming ever more manifest in the bigger cities: poverty, prostitution, diseases, and other afflictions. In the United States, the workers in these Urban Missions were known as the "friendly visitors". They were paid by the Church and other welfare organizations. Their work consisted of saying prayers for the troubled people they visited, teaching people about Christianity (teaching literacy—to read Bible). The idea here was to bring some relief to the people who suffered from so many social problems (Huff, D. 2008). The Preachers and ministers of the churches were very much in charge of the Urban Missions and urban missionaries.

Certain social problems captured the attention of the public. For instance, prostitutes during this period of time did not go unnoticed. Daily, in newspapers in New York and London, articles appeared about the dreadful state of the lives of the ladies who lurked in dark corners on the streets. Rescue societies were initiated with the purpose of finding a better way to help prostitutes. In the midst of all the caterwauling about the heinous evils of prostitution, a new philosophy of "scientific welfare" appeared, that claimed that the welfare of the disenfranchised should be, "secular, rational and empirical." This notion ran contrary to the orthodox idea about the Poor, which it was the duty of Christians to take care of the poor (Huff, D., 2008). By the end of 1800, a new system had evolved which focused on the cause of poverty. However, it was not enough to know the cause of poverty. Knowing its cause would not end it. Thus, poverty was something that had to be eliminated, and hence the Reform, Investigation and Residency movements came into being (Huff, D. 2008). These movements offered a variety of services that included education, legal aid and medical services. These services also advocated for changes in social administration. The administrators of these community movements became interested in the culture of the people that they wanted to help (Huff, D., 2008).

In the United States, the different methods of social work brought a fundamental question to the foreground: *Is Social Work a Profession?* This debate has its origin in the beginning of the 20th century, between the Society Organization of Welfare started by Mary Richmond, and the Community

Home Movement of Jane Addams. On one side of the debate were those who thought social problems should be examined in a scientific manner. These were the Mary Richmond advocates. However, there were the Jane Addams advocates who thought that helpers should actually live with those they helped. Therefore, traditional lines between interviewer and those helped should be eliminated (Parker, O. & Demiris, G., 2006).

Even though several Social Work Schools were opened and were formalized (accredited by states), the question about the stance of the social worker (interviewer) continued. In 1915, during the National Conference of Welfare and Corrections, Dr. Abraham Flechner discussed again the same question: Is Social Work a profession? Dr. Flechner made the claim that social work contained specialized knowledge. Flechner said that in its application of specific theories and intellectual knowledge, social work had the capacity to solve human and social problems (Lubove, 1965). This claim and others like it contributed to the professionalization of social work, which by now had divided the social worker's time between *Case work,* and adherence to scientific method . . . Notions of social work being rooted in Christianity were slowly eroding. The civil, secular society was out distancing well meaning Christians.

One: More on the Origins of Social Work

Social work, because it started with society's efforts to fight poverty, it was not long before politicians realized that poverty in a society bore negative consequences. Once the poor became an "issue' for politicians, social work became linked to the new idea of social welfare. Even though the concept of social welfare also goes back in time, and even though the practice of helping the poor has its roots in many civilizations and religions around the world, still, social welfare is a decidedly modern idea (Leiby, J., 1979).

The first friendly *visitors* were women who were volunteers or missionaries. The majority of them were from *high society*. These women put effort into reducing the poor's public burden through direct services and prayers. The friendly visitors studied and investigated the applications for help. Later, the applicants were separated into different classes: those that deserved help and those that did not deserve help. Friendly Visitors helped also by giving emotional support to the poor. They referred the poor with so many different problems to different places for assistance. One of the interesting outcomes of the Friendly Visitors was the following: for the first time members of high society were now intermingling with members of the lowest society. As this association continued between the very rich and the very poor, the rich could not help to make the comparison between their luxurious lives and the hard lives of the people they attempted to help. Women from the leisure class heard about a whole new world that they did not know existed. They heard about the abuses endured by the poor from their cruel employers. They heard about the dreadful and dangerous working conditions. It turned out that the notion that the poor were poor because they were morally defective turned out to not be true. The friendly visitors started to see poverty as a more complex problem than what they had originally hypothesized (Leiby, J., 1979).

While the attitudes of administrators and welfare organizations had changed, this changed the attitudes of the friendly visitors. The friendly visitors started to feel the need to be more professional. Emotionality expressed over the horrors of poverty and other social problems helped no one in the end. Thus, there was a general agreement amongst the friendly visitors that they needed more training that would help them to look at each case in a more objective fashion. In 1891, the Welfare Organizational Movement of New York started to publish and to implement new ideas in the field of social welfare. Training Programs under the direction of Mary Richmond (1861-1928), also a Friendly Visitor, were given around the country. Mary Richmond was a pioneer in the use of what would become social case work theory. Richmond believed in the relationship between people and their social environment as the major factor of their life situation or status. Her ideas were based on social theory and that social problems for a family or individual should be looked at by first looking at the individual or family, then including their closest social ties such as families, schools, churches, jobs, etc. Given this theory, now there was a legitimate way for a professional to intervene in the life of a poor person in need of assistance.

In 1898 these activities of Mary Richmond and others like her culminated in the establishment of a Summer School for Applied Philanthropy. After the establishment of the Summer School, the friendly visitors were replaced by what became: professional social workers. At the beginning the newly educated and trained friendly visitors identified themselves as "Social Workers." Soon, the first real social workers expanded their territory; it was not just the poor that would be their special concern. They would make child welfare and juvenile justice a part of their expertise. By the start of the 20th century, these new case workers were on the job, trying to improve the lives of a number of different kinds of people (Barker, R. 1998 and Wolf, L., 2002).

It turns out that that first Summer School mentioned above convened at Columbia University, which is still regarded as the school that offers the most premier program in Social Work in the whole United States. Since these first classes in 1898, social workers have been instrumental in developing organizations that pertain to social welfare, which exist in order to help people in need. Social workers, to this day, just as they did many years ago continue not only to place emphasis on social needs, but they help to highlight the very social problems that continue to plague the nation.

Two: American History

Modern social work in the United States has its origin in massive immigration witnessed in the beginning of the 19th century. Millions of new immigrants arrived in New York, from Russia, Poland, Ireland, and Germany. With new immigrants came new conglomerations of new social problems. New diseases also arrived in New York (Gehlert, S. & Brown, T.A., 2006). As the city became more congested and filled up with the newcomers, the newcomers picked up their suitcases and set out for other cities across the country. With the new immigrants, once again, came so many problems, like problems that pertained to health, or lack of health.

Elizabeth Blackwell was the first woman to practice medicine in the United States. She founded in 1853 the first

Medical Dispensary for women and indigent children (Elston, MA., 2004, 2008). The Medical Dispensary offered help to poor communities on the east side (NYC), and soon after it expanded beyond basic nursing. It began to provide people with real social evaluations of problems. The Dispensary offered also support to families of the area. In 1889, Jane Addams, a medical student, created something called: the Home for New Comers and Poor Communities in Chicago. The Home was a center that offered social services to the community. However, there was also a program for social research. Thus, it turns out that the founders of modern social work can trace their origins to this very Medical Dispensary of Elizabeth Blackwell, for it was not long before so called health professionals began to work with issues that pertained to social health problems (Gheler, S. & Brown TA., 2006).

Three: English History

The development of social work in England, as a discipline and profession, runs parallel to American history. Many people left the English country side to go to the industrial cities that promised employment in the new factories. The Industrial Revolution fueled the exeunt from the land to the cities, but no one could have foreseen the heinous living conditions that would be the result of this mass exodus. Cities like Manchester in the North of England and home to owners of large factories that employed workers in the manufacture of wool, teemed with poor children working long hours (18 hours per day), as well as young girls for the first time without husbands. Housing conditions were crowded and dirty. Diseases were rife. Infant mortality rate was extremely high. Drunks on the streets abounded. Robbers and thieves lurked in the doorways, and jumped when they could on the naïve young people arriving from the countryside.

The first social workers were called "Almoners" of hospitals, for these social workers worked in hospitals. The Free Royal Hospital hired Mary Stewart (who was the first almoner in 1895). Mary Stewart's role was to evaluate those people who sought attention from the hospital, and to make sure that they were considered "worthy" of free treatment. Soon, after the role of evaluator developed, this helped to usher in other social programs that were deemed valuable. By 1905, many other hospitals in London had developed functions similar to the Free Royal Hospital. In a way, what became the Counsel Almoners of the hospital system became also the standard for the new profession of Social Work. The Counsel of Almoners ended up supervising the fledging discipline of Social Work (Gheler, S T & Bronw, T., 2006)

Four: Social Work in Hospital Settings in the United States

In 1905, Social Work entered the hospitals in the United States at the invitation of Dr. Richard Clark Cabot, Chief of the Department of Medicine at Massachusetts General Hospital. While Dr. Cabot is known to have advanced clinical Hematology experience, he also turned out to be an innovator in methods of teaching. He was a definite pioneer in social work (Ghelert, S. & Brown TA., 2006). For example, Cabot created one of the first social work positions in the world, giving it to Garmet, Pelton, who later became sick with tuberculosis and had to retire. Next, that same position was given to Ida Cannon (Davidson, K. 1998 & Beder, J., 2006). What many people do not know is the hospital administrators had refused to hire social workers. Therefore, Cabot had to pay salaries out of his own pocket. Seven years later, because the filled social work position proved so successful, an actual social work specialty was established by the School of Social Work in Boston. Soon, several hospitals, mainly in the Northeast of the country established departments of social work.

Ida Cannon at Massachusetts General Hospital stayed in the position of Director of the Social Work Department forforty years (Barker, R., 1998). However, after 1905, many of the social workers were trained as nurses. Cabot changed the way that the department of ambulatory services of the hospital functioned, thinking that the social, economical, family and psychological conditions were the cause of many maladies that patients presented when they arrived to the hospital. Cabot thought that the social workers could work in a complementary relationship to the physicians, who would take care of the physiological problems, while the social workers would take care of the psychosocial problems. Besides this, Cabot also thought that the social worker could improve medicine by giving it a new perspective, which focused attention on care within the hospital setting (Beder, J., 2006)

In 1917, Cabot took a break to occupy a position on a Medical Reserve Team for one year. Later, he returned to Massachusetts General Hospital in 1918. In 1919, he took the position of President of the Ethics Department at Harvard University. During this time the hospital agreed to pay the salary of the social workers, for until that time Cabot had been paying the salary of thirteen social workers during a twelve year period. Later, when Cabot retired, he wrote about his experiences in a book entitled: Social Work (Cabot, R C., 1919).

In 1918, something called: The National Association of Hospital Social Workers (NASHW) was established. Its purpose was to improve the relationship between formal education and practice in hospitals. The role of the social worker during this time was to provide social services to people in need. Hospital administrators were adversarial, as they only wanted social workers in hospitals to evaluate the needs of patients seeking so called medical relief. However, patients at this time needed protection from the hospital itself, which picked and chose which patients to abuse. Poor patients were easy to abuse ((Davidson, K., 1998).

By 1929, there were ten university courses in medical social work. During this time, Psychiatry and Psychology started to compete with Social Work, to have social workers removed from the hospitals. Social work was able to adapt, however, and this is probably the major reason that the field of social work began to join in the rally around various psychological theories. One such theory was called Psychoanalysis. Because social work as a discipline was bent towards surviving, it began to be less interested in the social problems and the medical problems of patients. While this adaptation has been criticized, still, by separating from social problems, social work added a scientific base to its armature, which means that now it could deal with patients on a "talk therapy basis", or a psychotherapy basis. Here, certain behaviors of patients (clients) were now seen as emotional problems, and thus were no longer viewed as moral defects.

By the end of the 1930s, social work as a profession and as a discipline had been transformed; it was viewed as a fundamental component of how society would deal with its social problems. (Barker, L.1998). Monies (tax dollars) could now be spent on developing curricular that would propel people into social work programs in accredited schools of social work. By the time World War II came to an end, there had been an increase in the number of trained social workers released into the workforce. Many of these social workers ended up having a variety of experiences in welfare programs and their counterparts (Barker, R. L. 1998). However, as social workers became more legitimate workers in welfare settings, their original presence in hospitals diminished.

What should be gleaned from Social Work's history is its very origins begin in hospitals. The need that was originally felt for social workers in hospitals is still a need very much felt. More hospital personnel have lost knowledge of social workers in the ER or in the ICU, or in other medical/critical care units. Social Workers today should devote time to keeping medical personnel and administrators informed about the significance of the social workers' unique interventions with patients and with families (Wrenn, K. & Cowless, L A., 2000). Gaining this acceptance by doctors and nurses, but especially administrators who are interested today in "discharge" plans, more than anything else will be challenging. This means that while the interventions that social workers perform should be accepted by medical personnel, often it is not accepted. This is in the face of a mountain of proof, that social work interventions in hospitals have a proven track record of being therapeutically effective. Contrary to the opinion of misguided hospital administrators, interventions performed by social workers in the hospital are three things: cost effective, therapeutically effective, and family effective. While hospital personnel in charge of budgets should never cut the budget for social workers on staff. It turns out that social workers provide help that is akin to the help that the doctor and or the nurse give, for without social workers in the hospital, disease prevails instead of ease. While it is hard to measure ease, it is sufficient to say that hospitals who do keep social workers on staff have a success rate with clients (citizens-patients) that cannot be pointed to in other non-social work hospitals.

There is the myth, or the prevailing feeling that anyone can be a social worker in the hospital. This is not true. A social work intervention requires great skill, and when bungled the result can be likened to a bad operation. When staff is not educated about the role of social workers in hospitals, both patients and families experience a level of consternation that cannot be measured quantitatively. Yet, the qualitative literature corroborates the idea that staff and personnel are the key to opening the doors of the hospitals, to many more social workers who should be made, once again, as integral part of every health care organization. Social work services should be provided to individuals, families and other inpatient groups; to populations of special groups, communities and special health and educational programs (NASW, 2002).

Five: The Social Worker in the Hospital Setting:

One: Communicates, putting emphasis in the communication between the medical personnel, patients, families, and makes sure that their needs are met.

Two: Provides emotional support (psychotherapy), with emphasis in psychosocial problems and emotional needs that the patients or families may have.

Three: Protects the rights of patients and their families; and makes sure that the hospital system provides high quality care.

Four: Makes sure that all available resources are the most adequate for patients and their families.

Five: Intercedes between patients, families and the medical personnel.

Six: Intervenes, between patients, families and the medical personnel.

Seven: Coordinates, ongoing services to patients and their families.

Eight: Educates, and transmits knowledge to the medical personnel, patients, families; teaching them about Patient Rights and Advanced Directives, including end-of life.

During many years, Social Work's literature has hooted out the clarion call: Social workers must, "demonstrate their effectiveness" if they want to keep their employment in the health care system. In the meantime, while social workers in hospitals might be attempting to justify their existence, at the same time, evidence keeps appearing in the literature that makes it abundantly clear that social work is not recognized as a key factor in the hospital setting. In 1998, Rher, H.; Blumenfield, S. and Rosenberg named the following barriers that keep social work from having a strong presence in the hospital setting:

One: Its association with poor people.
Two: Its perception as a rival of the medical profession.

Three: Its lack of success demonstrating cost effectiveness of services provided.

Four: It is seen as ineffective in solving social problems (which requires a skill-set beyond the skill-set of the typical social worker

Five: Its lack of data to develop "better practice," as well as the lack of efficient collaboration with the other health care professionals to treat social health problems and its lack of "keeping records" of work in order to improve public health policy.

For a very long time it was concluded that the role of the social worker was better delineated by the Department of Social Work in the hospitals (Auslander, G. K., 2000), but that changed at some point in time. The entire reason d-etre for social workers in hospitals was being vigorously challenged. At first, the challenge came from hospital comptrollers in charge of budgets. Social workers in hospitals, while they delivered plenty of relief to patient and family, they did not help to generate financial gain. A surgeon removing a gall bladder can tag a quick $30,000 for the hospital. A sixteen year old male with a history of violence, with a gunshot wound in the head, with a distraught single mother of three other children is not a good script for generating funds for the hospital. While the social worker once delivers relief, it is not financial relief, and thus it eventually was deemed: "no relief at all." In the last seventy five years, social workers, even though their fledging beginnings were hospital related, have been eradicated from hospital staff across the country.

Doctors of Medicine, Nursing staff, and Psychiatrist, have a vague idea of what social workers do in the hospital setting.

When surveyed, they respond that the job of the social worker is mysterious, vague, and/or dangerous. Some health professionals flagrantly say: "they have no idea what a social worker does in the modern hospital." Oddly, social workers have a firm grasp of what doctors, nurses, psychiatrists and psychologists do. In a way, it would not be off the mark to dub social work as the invisible profession.

Social workers in hospital settings need to educate the medical staff, and administrators about their contribution to patient and family care. Education will help to emphasize not only the contents and purpose of the social worker's intervention in different areas of the hospital, but help to precisely lay out a specific skill-set that belongs to the social worker only, and to no other worker in the hospital. Interventions made by the social worker in the hospital are vital; these interventions cannot be dismissed or eradicated on the grounds of cost efficiency. After all, it is cost efficient to eradicate all social programs. The budget of the United States could be under control in a few years instead of thirty years, but no serious politician would make such a proposal. It would be career suicide. Yet, everyday, hospital staff members stand up in meetings and draw exit lines through social work staff. That one social worker now must be looking for a new job.

Social workers ought to demonstrate their skill-set in concrete terms, so all can understand that the training of a social worker cannot be duplicated by the doctor or the nurse, or the physical therapist, or the psychiatrist. This presentation and break-down of skill-set performance would definitely silence the naysayers. For instance, social workers, more than any other of the hospital personnel have been exposed to the latest communication theories that embrace "systems" and the need for the "system to remain open. Social workers can lead the way when it comes to hospital organization, and the need to eradicate hierarchical structures that glaringly obtrude, and therefore interfere with delivering the best services to consumers and families.

In the meantime, social workers must do their part as well, by providing hospital personnel with fact based evidence that evaluates: all interventions used by social workers in hospitals, assess relationships between all personnel, as well as examine social work practice, step by step, to see how better planning can return the social work profession to its former place, ensconced in the hospital setting. There is a single reason for this reentry into a hospital setting. Often, the disenfranchised are left behind in marginal places in society; they need to get settled however, inside of the margins of the society. The social worker working inside the hospital can keep the poor, for example, from being skirted to the outer perimeters of every community. In the end, one thing is certain, however, and that is a hospital without social workers is a hospital made for profit only. For profit as the only measurement in our mainline institutions today proves a dismal failure in the long run. Sometimes it is hard to count the worth of something like social workers on hospital staff, but when social workers are missing, as they have been in the last thirty years, this leaves a hole that can turn into a crater, which is no small indentation on the surface of the road ahead.

Six: Social Work in Mental Health

Because of the exeunt of social workers in hospitals, social workers had to find new roles for themselves. They decided to enter areas of mental health, and make themselves useful in this regard. This promotion of social workers in mental health has a history, just like the expulsion of social workers also has a history (National Institute of Mental Health, 1991). From Psychiatric Hospitals to the development of Community Centers, social workers have found themselves providing psychotherapy (counseling) to individuals and families. Also, social workers have been active in the actual prevention of mental illness. They have made efforts to develop public programs and allocate funds, to make sure that mental illnesses are treated with the same degree of gravity as medical illnesses.

By working with other health care professionals engaged in their practice, (i.e. psychologists and psychiatrists), social workers began to collaborate in the development of theories of Etiology and interventions, which have been now tried, modified and redefined through social work practice, and social work research. However, unbeknown to the unsuspecting investigator, emphasis on mental health instead of the effects of the social environment has changed the historical course of the typical social worker. Instead of the individual and his social environment, the social worker seeks to justify practice on the same grounds as the doctor or nurse, who subscribes to the bio-psychosocial approach to the consumer. This may seem like a small detail in a large panoramic view of the place of the social worker in society, but actually it is not a small gnat or flies in the ointment.

Now, the social workers work on the psyche of the individual, helping him/her to find happiness, peace inside of him, herself. The consumer's social environment has fallen by the historical wayside.

The main objective of social workers in Mental Health is to be able to help people who suffer from mental illness, so that they can function in the world in which they live. This new adopted role of the social worker has helped to ameliorate the conditions for the mentally ill, who are no longer locked up in mental institutions. The concept subscribed to now be: the social worker helps the consumer "adjust" to the realities of life (National Institute of Mental Health, 1991).

The social worker today, even though he/she may not show up in his/her place of origin, the hospital, still, he/she shows up in psychiatric hospitals and Mental Health Clinics. Social workers also work in prisons, court houses, schools, and social programs. Presumably, unlike psychiatrists, the social worker is trained to be interested in treating the whole person. Yet, these new adopted roles and environments for the social worker is challenging, for the medical model is hard to squash. It prevails, and this means that the social worker's training to treat the whole person bumps head-on into psychiatry's focus, which is to cure the illness by prescribing psychotropic medication (National Institute of Mental Health, 1991). What this really means is even the adopted role of the social worker, to be the advocate for mental health, has also been challenged as well. The typical social worker in a psychiatric facility or a mental health clinic has his/her hands tied by the psychiatrist who does not really believe that psychotherapy conducted by a social worker helps the patient as much as an anti-psychotic medicine. If this is true, it might have been wiser for the social worker to remain in the hospital, where becoming an orphan to be adopted was not an option.

Additional Considerations:

In order to understand the origin and development of the Social Work profession, one could hurry back in time, back before the 19th century, all the way to the 17th century in England. There are those scholars who argue that it was at this time in England that the bases of Social Welfare were actually established for the creation of social services. Changing relations between the King, the nobility, the merchants, and the peasants was shifting in England.

England was different than other European countries, because let us remember that way back in the 13th century, King John was forced to sign the Magna Carta, which was a document that teamed the nobility with the merchants and the people . . . against the King. In other words, of all the European countries, it was the English that wanted to limit the power of the King, for in France and Russia the nobility teamed up with the ruler against the regular people. By limiting the power of the King, the English were the first people to think about the well being of the commoners. This is what is meant by "social welfare, for social welfare and a concept of social welfare springs forth from the common welfare or the common people, or the regular people, who were always in the majority.

If one wanted to look further at the professionalization of social work, one would have to visit the work of Flexner and

Greenwood, who make the aforementioned claim, that social welfare was the springboard for social services. Yet, the authors also make the claim that in order for social work to be regarded as a legitimate profession, it has to adhere to the following criteria. Greenwood, contrary to Flechner (NASW, 2002), concluded that social work is a profession because it espouses specific guidelines.

1. Has systematic body of theories that support what it does
2. Has professional authority that results from theory
3. Has community knowledge that the profession is valid
4. Has a code of ethics which regulates the behavior of its members, has a professional culture consistent with a vocabulary and professional methodology.

Social work is a profession and academic discipline engaged in the promotion of social wellbeing, social changes and social practice. This profession works towards the reach and practice to improve the quality of life of each individual, groups, and communities in society. Social workers develop interventions thru research, administration, ongoing communication, direct practice and education. Research is often focused in areas such as human development, social administration, public administration, evaluation of programs and community developments. Social workers are organized in professional local, national, continental and international groups. Social work is an interdisciplinary field that includes economics, education, sociology, medicine, philosophy, anthropology and psychology (NASW, 2002).

Social work is based upon the diverse knowledge that comes from research and evaluation of practice, including its own knowledge of specific contents. Also, social work acknowledges the complexity of the interactions between people and the environment, and the ability of individuals to cope with multiple psychosocial problems. Social work as a profession takes from other theories of human development, social theory and social systems theories, in order to analyze complex situations and structures. Social workers seek to improve individual challenges, social and individual organizations (Definition of Social Work, 2000).

For more than a century, the social work profession has developed and reinvented itself; it has responded to social and economic changes. Yet, upon further investigation, social work has managed to keep its unique description. It works to relieve the needs of the most vulnerable of the society. Today, social workers constitute a large number of professionals that work in areas of health and mental health, the educational system, justice system; they provide services for families of different ethnic and cultural groups, as well as services for geriatric citizens in Nursing Homes (NASW, 2002).

REFERENCES

Barker, Robert L. (1998). Milestones in the development of Social Work and Social Welfare. Washington, DC. NASW

Beder, J. Hospital Social Work: The interface of Medicine and caring. Routlege: New York.

Cabot, R.C. (1919). Social work, Webpage: Google-Books-dsC.

Davidson, K. (1998). Role Blurring and the social Worker's search for a clear domain. Health and Social work, 15, 228-234 meeting in Montreal, Canada. International federation of Social Workers, 04-10-05 retrieved 2008.

Elston, M. A (2004)-2008). Blackwell, Elizabeth (1821-19100. Oxford. Dictionary of National Biography, Oxford University Press.

Gehler, S. A. T. A Browne (2006). Chapter Two: The Conceptual Underpinning of Social in Health Care. Handbook of Health Social Work. New Jersey: WILEY.

Huff, D. (2008). Chapter I. "Scientific Philanthropy" (1860-1900). The Social Work History Station. Boise State University. P. 02-20

Huff, D. (2008). Chapter I-II "Missionaries & Volunteers." The Social Work History Station. Boise State University Press.

Huff, D. (2008). "Chapter II Settlements" (1880-1900). The Social work History Station. Boise State University. P. 02-20

Leiby, J. (1979). A History of Social Welfare and Social Work in the United States, New York: Columbia University Press.

Lubobe, R. (1965). The Professional Altruism. The Emergence of Social Work as a Career, 1890-1930, Cambridge, MA Harvard University Press.

National Institute of Mental Health. (1991). Building Social Work Knowledge for Effective Services and Policies. Washington, DC: Author.

Parker-Oliver, Debra; Demiris, George (2006). "Social Work Informatics: A New Specialty." Social Work. National Association of Social Workers (NASW) %1 (2): 127-134

Rher, H., Blumenfield, S. & Rosenberg, G. (1998). Creative Social Work in Health Care: Clients, \the community, and organization. New York: The Mount Sinai Medical Center. Press.

Woolf, Linda M. (2002). Women's Intellectual Contribution to the Study of Mind and Society; Mary Ellen Richmond. Webster University Press.

CHAPTER TWO

Social Work Interventions in the Hospital Setting

I T IS IMPORTANT FOR social workers in the hospital setting to demonstrate to the medical staff (Doctors/Nurses), and administrators that the various interventions they make in the different units of the hospital are of great value, for social workers were and remain an integral part of every health care organization (NASW, 2002). Social workers should be at the disposal of individuals, families, and other groups; to people of special groups, communities, and to special programs in health care education (NASW, 2002). It is my strong opinion that social workers placed in the hospital setting provide *concrete* services as well as *clinical services*; they assist patients and their families to overcome a crisis: admittance to the hospital, sudden death of a loved one, domestic violence, child and elderly abuse, alcohol and drug abuse, homelessness, mental illness; as well as issues that pertain to discharge planning.

Concrete Services; are those services that revolve around the information and activities of the referrals made by the medical staff. These include connecting patients with available resources; for example assisting in the coordination of services of admission and discharge from the hospital, attention to families of patients during their admission, helping with transportation services and getting personal assistance and medical supplies.

Concrete Services:

1. Eligibility for social services.
2. Helping patients with getting medical equipment.
3. Interpreting patient's feelings to the medical staff.
4. Explain medical orders to patients.
5. .Mediating between patients and the medical staff.
6. Explaining hospital services to the community.
7. Management of discharge planning from the hospital.
8. Referral to patients to community support services.
9. Counseling patients about following medical recommendations.
10. Working with families to understand the patient's medical condition, and offer community support services at home.

Clinical Services; are the different forms of counseling (psychotherapy) that deal with interpersonal relations between the social worker, the patient and the family. The focus here is in attitudes, feelings, perceptions, decisions or behaviors of the patient or families. Frequently such services have to do with problems of patients and families in relation to their adaptation and acceptance to the services offered by the hospital (diagnosis, prognosis, and treatment plans).

Clinical Services:

1. Collaboration with the health care professionals.
2. Diagnosis of psychosocial problems.
3. Recommend psychiatric treatment.
4. Help patients to overcome emotional crisis.
5. Give emotional support to patients and their families.
6. Offer information to families about illness, symptomatology and medication.
7. Offer information to patients and families about the importance of taking medication regularly and side effects.
8. Help patients to adapt to illness, understand the symptoms and how to manage them effectively.
9. Use of psychotherapy techniques.
10. Provide psychotherapy to patients and families with emotional problems.
11. Educate health care professionals about social services.
12. Consult with health care professionals about patients with psychosocial problems.

Social Work Intervention in the Emergency Room; is a non-traditional specialty that involves working with physicians and nurses who are more attuned to illness and trauma than to patient's social needs (Elliot, M.,1987). The social worker in the ER collaborates with physicians, nurses and other medical staff to identify the psychosocial needs of patients and their families, not just the presenting problem. The social worker contributes to the overall effectiveness of the operation of the ER by helping patients and their families cope with their crisis, including but not limited to sudden death, homelessness, alcohol/substance abuse, mental illness, child abuse, elder abuse, victims of domestic violence, sexual abuse, as well as with issues of goals of care, advance directives, palliative care, and discharge planning. Patients are admitted either as a result heart attack, stroke, drug related poisoning, pneumonia, major trauma as a result of road traffic accidents, falls, burns, and industrial accidents or violence.

Social Work Intervention in the Intensive Care Unit; as well as in the ER, is a non-traditional specialty. In the ICU, the social worker collaborates with the medical staff in identifying patients' and families psychosocial problems, helping them to have the opportunity to ask questions, to express their feelings, fears, helping them to overcome the crisis, providing emotional support, as well as with issues of health care decisions and medical care. The social worker in the ICU is constantly challenged to demonstrate the value of his/her interventions with patients and families. The social worker helps families to overcome crisis, trauma, death of a loved one, and should be prepared to evaluate those needs and intervene accordingly.

Social Work Intervention in the Medical-Surgical Unit/ Pulmonary Unit (Discharge Planning); generally implies working with other systems outside the hospital setting, including referrals to services in the community (home care services, skilled nursing facilities, alcohol and rehabilitation programs, homeless shelters, etc.). Some patients need personal care at home; medical supplies (wheelchairs, walkers, crutches, etc). Other patients may not have financial resources or medical insurance to pay for their medical bills, the social worker makes referrals to the designated department of the hospital for financial assistance and application for emergency medical coverage.

The Social Worker in the Hospital Setting:

1. **Communicates;** putting emphasis on communication between the medical staff, patients and their families, and makes sure that patient's needs are met.
2. **Provides emotional support;** with emphasis to the psychosocial and emotional needs of patients and their families.
3. **Protects patients' rights;** making sure that the hospital system provides high quality services to patients and their families.
4. **Makes sure;** that the available resources for patients and their families are adequate.
5. **Advices;** and personalizes interactions, understands feelings, attitudes and behaviors of patients and their families.
6. **Intervenes;** between patients, families and the medical team.
7. **Coordinates;** organizing services for patients and families.
8. **Educates;** and transmits knowledge to others, teaching topics about Advanced Directives, including end of life issues.

Review of the literature about social work interventions in the hospital setting since 1967 to the present, demonstrates that there is still not enough knowledge about social work interventions in the in the Emergency Room, Intensive Care Units, and Medical Surgical Units. The efficient use of social workers depends mostly on how other health care professionals perceive the practice of social work. Those outside the profession may not be familiarized with the variety of services and skills that are provided by social workers. The hospital system may limit social workers to provide concrete services (eligibility for social services, helping patients to obtain medical supplies, make telephone calls, finding clothes, care fare for transportation, among others.), but keep them from being able to use their clinical skills: to help patients overcome the emotional impact of illness or hospitalization. Lack of knowledge of what social workers do in the hospital setting, however, ends up causing conflict also with other professionals and their ability to collaborate with social workers. This is foolhardy, for doctors and social workers are in the hospital to help the patient recover.

Social workers in the hospital setting need to be able to provide certain clinical interventions; they aid in patient health care education. Social workers engage in clinical practice decisions and ameliorate ethical dilemmas. Social workers encourage consumer (patient) diversity. Yet, there is a need for more social work research, which explores in depth the need to reexamine what social workers do in the hospital setting.

Because hospital-based social work is not typically income generating, social work departments have been vulnerable to downsizing and elimination. Where social work services have been retained, most time is spent in negotiating with managed care companies, or providing concrete services for patients, such as arranging transportation, obtaining medical equipments, home care services, skilled nursing homecare, medical coverage, clothing, or making telephone calls.

Social work in the hospital setting refers both, to *direct practice,* which is based on face to face interactions with patients and families, and *indirect practice,* which involves interactions with agencies and community support systems. Those outside the social work profession may not be familiar with the range of services and skills provided by social workers. The health care delivery system may limit social work to provide only concrete services and fail to utilize the social worker's skills in helping patients and families cope with the emotional impact of illness and hospitalization.

For years, literature in the field of social work in the hospital setting has called for social workers to demonstrate their effectiveness, so they can retain their position in the field of social work in the hospital. Yet, there is evidence that social work should be recognized as a key factor in smooth hospital operations. Rher, H & Blumenfield, S. (1998) indicated that the following factors are barriers which prevent social work from having a solid position in the health care systems in hospitals:

1. Its association with relatively poor people.
2. The perception as rival with the medical staff.
3. The lack of success demonstrating cost-effectiveness in providing services.
4. Is seen as ineffective in solving social problems (which requires the power of other than social work).

5. Lack of data to develop "better practice," as well as the failure in applying process for administration, lack of collaboration with other professionals to treat social health problems; and its lack of "keeping record" of the work to improve public social health policy.

Social work entered to the hospitals in the United States by invitation of Dr. Richard Cabot, Chief of Medicine at Massachusetts General Hospital in Boston, in 1905. Cabot created one of the first social work positions in the world, giving it to Garmet Pelton and later to Ida Cannon (Davidson, K. 1998 & Beder, J. 2006). After seven years of having created the service, a medical social work position was established by the School of Social Work of Boston. Several hospitals in the north eastern part of the country established social work departments. Cannon remained in the social work position at the Massachusetts General Hospital for forty years. She became the Director of the Department of Social Work (Barker, R. 1998). After 1905, the majority of social workers were trained as nurses (the first social workers were women). The role of the social worker at that time was to provide social services to people in need, however, the hospital administrators only wanted social workers to evaluate and alleviate the medical (only medical) needs of patients, and, prevent abuse of the patients by the hospital itself (Davidson, 1998). Cabot came along and profoundly changed the way that the ambulatory services of the hospital were functioning. He said that the economic conditions of the family were problematic, along with the many psychological manifestations of patients. This sounds mundane now and a firm grasps of the obvious, but for the times it turns out that

Cabot was a true pioneer. No one else was thinking about social work in the way he thought about it. One thing is for sure; he roots social work and all of its many facets in a hospital setting.

Cabot believed social workers could work in collaboration with the physicians who were taking care of the medical (physiological) problems of patients, and the social workers would take care of the social problems. Cabot also thought that social work could improve Medicine, giving medicine a new perspective on care within the confines of the hospital (Davidson, K. 1998). There is no doubt that Cabot was out to expand on the role of the social worker, for once the social worker was placed in hospital a myriad number of roles were added to social work in general.

In 1917 the National Social Workers' Exchange was formed with the purpose of improving the connection between formal education and practice in hospitals. The Exchange dealt with a number of issues including employment, working conditions, and salaries. The success of the exchange provided evidence that there was a need for a national organization. By 1920, school social service programs were functioning in Iowa, Massachusetts, and New York. In 1921 a group from the Social Workers' Exchange met at the National Conference and voted to change their name to the American Association of Social Workers (Barker, R., 1998).

For many years it was concluded that the social work roles were better performed by the department of social work within the hospital (Auslander, G K., 2000). However, in several places around the world, this logic was questioned. Because hospital social work departments did not generate income, some had to be downsized or eliminated.

As mentioned by Davidson, K. (1998) and Cowles, L. A (2000), social work in hospital settings has developed its own unique knowledge base; it has influenced patient care, as well as promotes the psychosocial component of medical care. The reason for the disagreement about the role of the social worker in the hospital setting is evident, for it is the expectations of other medical care professional and how they view social work and social workers that is keeping collaboration between all professionals from going forward.

The medical work and the hospital cannot be like a medieval fiefdom divided into separate domains that never overlap or intermingle. Doctors and nurses and administrators must recognize the unique contributions of the social worker in the hospital that the job is not just about the provision of concrete services. Doctors can no longer maintain their bureaucratic stance, ensconced in their ivory towers built upon layers of hierarchical dominance that no longer provides the best care or actual wellness for the patient. Nurses have rebelled against the superiority and arrogant behaviors of the doctors, and now it is time for the social workers to do the same. Social workers in hospitals want more independence, which means they do not want their skill-set to be relegated to the irrelevant pile. Slowly, we are inching towards an intense examination of this skill-set, but it is safe to say that no other professional in the hospital can do what the social worker can do for the patient.

Currently, colleagues in the fields of medicine, nursing, psychiatry, and psychology only have a vague idea of what social workers do. In some instances, they say that what social workers do is difficult, but it is also labeled "mysterious" and even "dangerous." In the long run, however, when surveyed or questioned in person, hospital personnel are not necessarily interested in what social workers do in hospitals; no explanation is important.

When the shoe is on the other foot, it turns out that social workers have knowledge of what doctors do, nurses, psychiatrics, and psychologists do. Social work ends up being an *invisible profession.*

Social workers often do little or nothing to promote their services. The skills, abilities and contributions are not evident to social workers themselves. For instance, the social worker may not know that it takes skill to be in a room with a suffering patient, even though the social worker has received years of training in and around the instance of being in a room with a patient who is experiencing intense physical pain. All the years of training, however, go to the wayside when the social worker is questioned further about his unique skill-set in this example of the suffering patient. This is odd; for doctors and nurses know what their skill set is in this instance of the suffering patient.

The social worker is communicating with the patient, for the patient may be dying and know that this is the case. That patient wishes to put his affairs in order; there are telephone calls to be made. The social worker might be interacting with the family of the patient, for the patient may be a victim of a violent crime, a random shooting. This intervention with family is complex. There is a mother and father and spouse and children, who all have needs in this crisis-ridden time. Only the social worker will know as much about the family and the sub-sets within this incredible system called a family, wherein one participant ends up having so much impact on another member of the family. In Systems Theory, only the social worker (possibly the nurse) will understand well that the recovery of one within a dysfunctional system will bring out dysfunction in a new member of the family. The petty thief in the hospital with a long criminal record going back to teen years may upon discharge from the hospital see "the light of day", but his younger brother will pick up the ball and run along with crime, in order to maintain the dysfunctional homeostasis of this particular family.

The social worker as a trained psychotherapist, working in the hospital setting is often dealing with intense emotions. Psychotherapeutic intervention is an art form. The ability to listen, think, advocate, mediate, consult, plan, teach, advise, improve, and make decisions about interventions are all precisely learned skills, that help to almost surgically remove obstacles and solve problems of patients and their respective families.

One of the major gripes with placing social workers in hospitals is it is not cost effective. However, a brief history of the profession of social work and its basic concepts demonstrate that many of the principles of social work are compatible with the mandate to deliver the highest quality services to patients for the lowest possible cost (Soskis, C. 1995 & Cowles, L A., 2000). This compatibility has to do with social workers themselves, being able to move patients through the hospital system in the most efficient ways. Without the presence of social workers in hospitals, costs invariably rise. Administrators appear puzzled by this rise in cost.

Effective, comprehensive discharge planning has been studied by social work researchers over the past two decades, especially since the effort has increased to shorten the stay of the patient, for every day in the hospital adds money to the bill. The average length of stay for hospitalization has been shortened by three days for all patients across all age groups. In the case of older patients, the stay has been decreased by seven days (Popovic, J. R. & Kozac, L. J., 2000). In response to shorter length of stay, past research suggest that the profession of social work has recognized early on that there were gaps in the knowledge shared by hospital and community based agencies charged with community care, gaps in information shared between providers, and gaps in knowledge of discharge education for patients and families.

Health care in the 21st century will prove to be very exciting, but especially as it pertains to social workers and the role they will play, must play in health care organizations, like hospitals. With the increase in the senior population, the newest biomedical advances, shortages of health care workers, ever-rising medical costs, along with the continuing healthcare disparities for minorities and women and children, combined with the dramatic increase in knowledge emanating from the newest information technologies, positions the social worker at a crossroads, or even a dangerous intersection. Do the profession and the professional follow the path of least resistance? Or does the social worker follow the path less followed, and speak out about the unique skill-set of the social worker. The social worker has the ability to impact health policies, as well affect patient care strategies and tactics in hospitals. The social worker can be the visionary, as she/he was the visionary in the beginning of the profession's history. Social workers can provide clinical leadership in the area of psychotherapy, as well as articulate the use of evidence-based theories, and, put them into practice. In fact, social workers the history and practice of social work since the year 1900 have been the inspiration for holistic human values and ethical principles, even in the field of medicine. Social workers have kept the doctors and nursing "caring", for caring for the one (individual) and the many (the group) has been the hallmark of the entire social work profession. These principles and adherence to value, however, was originally worked out in hospitals, which are nothing more than care centers for the whole person. The encroachment of the medical, chiseling down the person to just biology and physiology, or simply diagnosis and treatment of the physical alone is not treatment of whole human beings. To de-compartmentalize man in this way is wrong. Social workers know it is wrong. They have always known it is wrong.

As a caring profession, social work has a unique opportunity to influence health care by advocating for the health and needs of others in society. Social work has adopted a social justice philosophy which strives to positively influence public policy for the welfare of the poor, sick, and vulnerable by maintaining its belief in the inherent dignity of the person. Social advocates influence society by giving voice to those suffering, and by changing social structures that do promote health and wellbeing. Responsibility for this change is best assumed by the social work profession, which historically has been positioned at the forefront of patient-centered care.

To move forward a health care system grounded in social justice principles, social workers must reflect on the rights of people by evaluating organizational structures for disparities, and working for long-term social change. Social workers need to effectively address gaps in health education, resources, and access. Social work as a profession focuses on the common good, thereby grounding the practice in respect for human dignity, solidarity, family, care for the poor and vulnerable, human equality and right to life, charity and justice, and active stewardship of resources. Social workers cultivate community and public participation in health and wellness. This is the true promotion of peace.

Conclusion and Recommendations:

Social workers in hospital settings need to educate the medical staff, administrators, and other health care professionals about their contribution to patient care and helping families. Social workers are the only ones who can efficiently work within the system to reach this challenging objective. Education will emphasize not only the content and purpose of the intervention of the social worker in different areas, it will also emphasize the social worker's skills and abilities to demonstrate and communicate their interventions. The social worker should use this educational platform to speak about the worth of social work interventions. Social work programs at the graduate level should seek to educate social workers on how to reach the ears of other medical health professionals, so that doctor and nurses do not remain ignorant. The entire "system" which includes the social worker, doctor and nurse is a constellation of "care" at every level of what it means to be human: physical, mental, and even spiritual [transcendent]. The fact is: Social workers with accurate and careful analysis of the boundaries of their work, who know the importance of their interventions, can establish a clear dominion for practice in the complex hospital system. There is no further need to be confused or befuddled by what social workers do in hospitals, or be mystified by their myriad interventions, each one crucial to the well being of the single patient and the multiple patients.

Social work interventions in the hospital settings, specially the Emergency Room, Intensive Care Units, and Medical Surgical Units, are a specialty which requires absolute explicit knowledge. We cannot allow this work to be implicit or assumed, or known by the name "intuitive" or "common sense" behavior. Social work interventions are specific skill-set that must be taught and learned.

Even though, research done by social workers in these above areas is limited, especially if they are compared with studies done by Medicine and Nursing, still, this does not mean that social work educators cannot change their minds. To this date, there have not been conducted empirical studies about the effectiveness of social work intervention in hospital settings. To this date, no one even has connected the dots historically, to show that social workers started in hospitals. There is no reason to push them to the periphery in today's world.

There is a need from social workers and the profession to clarify their role and clarify what is meant by "intervention." This is a crucial task; nothing can be done until this is done. How can the social work profession as it is practiced in hospitals be realized as important until social workers as a group write their own policy statements about the nature of intervention, the limits and the extent of intervention. First, social workers must define their role, and they can do this by harkening back to their won valued history. Next, they can name the interventions, one by one, and if the name is and needs updating, then so be it. This does not mean that social workers give up their values, all because they become explicit about their role in the hospital and kinds of interventions for which they are responsible, and have always been responsible.

Last, based on social justice principles, social work has a duty to advocate for reinventing the discharge planning process, as there are vast disparities in this process. The patient is not always being discharged with his/her best interest in mind. Often the discharge is predicated on the number of hospital beds that need to be filled and filled again a few days later. The number of hospital beds available or not available cannot be arranged on an assembly line/industrial model. We cannot push a button and get rid of a patient. Yet, today this may be the very case. By using social justice principles embedded in sound discharge planning, this system change project could recommit the entire staff in hospital to a new level of concern, care, and cure. This new commitment or recommitment could transcend the walls of the health care institutions and filter itself into the interstices of society itself (Hager, J. S., 2010)

Recommendations for Further Research:

1. **Intervention Development;** research should move toward development of model interventions as well as addressing the organization as well as identification of structural barriers for social work to their implementation within.

2. **Systems Coordination;** better communication and coordination of services are needed between social workers and medical staff in the hospital setting.

3. **Engagement of Clients;** development of effective outreach and transitional services to individuals and families are essential, given the challenges of working with those who are severely ill, resistant to treatment, multi-systems users, persons with different socio-cultural backgrounds, and psychosocial problems.

4. **Measurement Issues;** new approaches to research design and measurement are needed to address target populations involved in the hospital setting to address the patient-social work dynamic (what occurs in the intervention process), and to address practice setting variation.

5. **Professional Collaboration;** social work researchers and practitioners should team up with researchers from other disciplines (Medicine, Nursing) in order to advance knowledge on social work interventions in the hospital settings

REFERENCES

Auslander, G.K. (2000). Outcome of social work Interventions in health care settings. Social Work in Health Care, 31 (2) 31-46

American fact Finder (2009). U. S. Census Bureau. Population estimates for New York State by Count-retrieved on July 2008.

Barker, R. L. (1998). Milestones in the Development Of Social Work and Social Welfare. Washington, DC NASW Press.

Beder, J. (2006). Hospital Social Work: The interface of Medicine and caring. Routlege: New York

Bronx Lebanon Hospital Center (2007). Department of Medicine. Bronx, New York: Author.

Elliot, M. (1987). Roles and functions of social work. Encyclopedia of Social Work. 18th ed. (pp.500-502) Washington, DC: NASW Press.

Cowles, L.A. (2000). Social work in the health field: A care perspective. New York: The Haworth Press.

Davidson, K. (1998). Role blurring and the social worker's search for a clear domain. Health and Social Work, 15, 228-234

Hager J. S. (2010). Effects of Discharge Planning Intervention on Perceived Readiness for Discharge. St. Catherine University.

Mizrahi, T., & Abramson, J. (2000). Collaboration between social workers and physicians: Perspectives on a share case. Social Work in Health Care (pp. 31-3).

National Association of Social Workers (2000). Code of Ethics of the National Association of Social Workers. Washington, DC: Author.

Popovic J. R. & Kozac L. J. (2000). National hospital discharge survey: Annual summary, 1998. Vital and health statistics No. 148. Hyattsville, MD: National Center for Health Statistics.

Rher, H., Blumenfield, S., & Rosenberg, G. (1098). Creative social work in health care: Clients, the community, and your organization. New York: The Mount Sinai Medical Center. Press.

Wrenn, K. & Rice, N. (1993). Social work services in the Emergency department: An integral of health care safety net. Academy of Emergency Medicine, I, 247-253. XVI.

CHAPTER THREE

Social Work and the Importance of Communication with Families of Patients Admitted To the Intensive Care Unit

P EOPLE GET NERVOUS AND anxious when a family member becomes ill and is admitted to the hospital Medical Intensive Care Unit (MICU). They fear mostly that the patient will die soon. The ICU social worker provides specifics kinds of help. He/she provides emotional support (psychotherapy), as well as assists the family in reaching an agreement with the kind of outcome they prefer. The social worker gives guidance and direction to the family, as he/she helps the family realize that their loved can recover, or least realized that the patient will probably recover.

The social worker helps families to express their feelings, so that final things they wish to say can be the kinds of things that will best be remembered if the patient does not recover. If the patient only has so long to live, then the social worker can help families make the best use of the time left. All along the way, the social worker is the main support for the family; it is not the nurse or the doctor. It is the social worker.

When people receive news of a final diagnosis that is not reversible, when no recovery is in sight, family members react in different ways that are often dissimilar. These dissimilar reactions can be surprising; the social worker must be prepared for the widest possible number of reactions. At the same time, the social worker helps families to adhere to the final wishes of the patient. If the patient did not have time to make out a list of final wishes, then the social work has the skill to broach the subject at this hour, so that all can come to an agreement how the patient will spend his/her final hours.

Even though the social worker has the skills to discuss all of these things with family members, this does not mean that all members will be able to proceed in a logical, rational, compassionate manner. There are so many factors to consider here: the patient's age, time with the illness (injury), and personality of the patient. These same factors apply to the family members as well, for they are of a certain age, and they too have been suffering for a certain amount of time with their loved one being ill or injured. It is hard to accept reality, and thus families become very depressed. Some family members will be able to get on with their lives, but there will always be one or two, a mother with a sick child, or wife with an injured husband who just cannot move away from the approaching death of their beloved. Here, the social worker is a grief counselor.

Sometimes fear accounts for the reaction of some family members. They are petrified; they cannot imagine their world without mother, or father, or their son or daughter. This is why some family members become very angry, even with the social worker or the doctor or the nurse. Others sink into a terrible depression, a veritable slough of despair, an abyss that is very deep and dark. There are the anxious types who check on the patient every two minutes, and there are the screamers who start yelling at the "incompetent" doctor who has killed their mother or killed their child."

All of these intense emotions must be sorted out and managed by the social worker. The social worker here is in charge of panic, insult, curses, and even in charge of the family members who storm out the door of the ICU, threatening to never return. The gunshot wound in their father's head is "just not their problem". Aguilera, D. C. & Messick, J. M. (1974) attributed the individual differences of family members to the following factors:

1. The individual perception to tensed events.
2. The availability of support systems.
3. The defense mechanisms used by people to cope with different events.

What is important for the social worker is to allow all family members to express themselves, not in any uniform way, but in the individual ways that suit them, their age and relationship to the patient, and their personality type. The social worker's intervention must fit the situation and fit the family member. However, what is crucial is the social worker remains next to the family and works as an advocate for every need, every voice, every pained interlude whatever it may be. Yes, there are many emotional needs here and they all must be met, but the social worker survives the storm by respecting the individual members of the unit, the family, and by understanding the dynamics as well of the family as a whole, or as a system. It does not sound like much, that the social worker gives assurance to all, but let us keep in mind that this assurance is individualized. It is not one assurance fits all; it is assurance that fits like a glove every single family member, and even fits the patient him/herself.

To the families dealing with a loved one in the ICU, let us remember that each member at heart believes that the patient will undoubtedly recover. This is what they all believe and must believe. Hoping for recovery is good; and this is why it is depressing and wrong to prepare family members for the worst. The worst will occur on its own; we do not need to predict the worst, which is death

Families, rather than being prepared for death, should be prepared for life, or be prepared to interact with the patient and with each other in particular ways that are very hopeful.

1. Spend more time with the patient, more than what the doctors have suggested.
2. Have more opportunities to go places that they always wanted to go with the patient.
3. Have more time to be able to express their wishes about medical care during end of life and to make funeral arrangements.
4. Have more time to be able to tell the patient the things that they always wanted to say but never did.
5. Have the opportunity to explore and understand the spiritual meaning of life and death.
6. Have the opportunity to tell the patient how important he/she was in their lives.
7. Have more time to share their wishes with other family members.
8. Have more days to feel better.
9. Have more time to simply enjoy the presence of those they love.

10. Be in peace with them, eschewing sorrow and replacing it with joy and gratitude . . . for the time that was left to them.

Good communication not only should depend on the social worker. However, often the social worker becomes a teacher, a teacher of good communication skills, as families are not good communicators. Certain kinds of highly charged connotative language can be ambivalent, causing misunderstandings that alarm the patient and alarm other family members as well. This is why the social worker and the patient and the family members can all end up on different pages. Sometimes the gap in misinterpreted meaning puts each player not just on a different page, but in a completely different book. In the meantime, the patient's needs are overlooked, for the patient and the families and the social worker are all firing on different communication cylinders.

When it is time for the social worker to tell the family that the illness of the patient is not curable, and that the risk of death is imminent, it is a very good idea to make sure that one is not standing in the hallway, or in front of the Coca Cola machine. The family should be seated in a comfortable room that is sound proof and private. Environment is important; it has an effect on all of us, but it especially has an effect on a stressed family. Therefore, standing in corridors or in the waiting area is not advisable. Taking the family to a private, comfortable room will have the best effect on the family; the psychological impact of the traumatic news will definitely be lessened.

Bad news can be ameliorated, toned down, and framed therefore in the best possible light. When the social worker has taken the time to understand the family dynamics, or the family's rhythm, then it will be that much easier to say what needs to be said about the patient and the fact that the patient will not recover from the illness or injury. All that is said should be said in an honest, direct, sensible manner. The social worker should stop at syncopated intervals to ask the family if they have any questions. Any and all questions should be carefully answered. Answering questions is an excellent technique for bringing family members out of denial, as they get to hear their own voice voicing the unthinkable, that their loved one will not recover. Yet, the social worker can always expect to see the family's sense of astonishment after bad news, as they are trying to piece together a story that they never thought they would hear. In the midst of this consternation, the social worker has the opportunity to probe through a lot of feelings that are not normally expressed, but only in this emergency.

It is important to schedule meetings with family members, as this proves an effective to discuss issues that pertain to the difficult decisions ahead. Clearly, at this point, often the most difficult decision pertains to whether treatment should cease. Even though the treatment is sometimes useless, because of lack of information families continue, and the process of dying becomes onerous. Families value the information shared by the social worker, but what they really value, once again, is the opportunity to ask questions. In the midst of all the questions, often the social worker realizes that family members are expressing deeper levels of grief; they are actually already mourning the loss of their loved one. The social worker offers the families so much emotional support at this time, that families send small gifts and cards for years to the worker, to thank him or her for their endurance and patience and incredible intelligence that led them through the valley . . . through the shadow of death.

Denial is the best defense mechanism that protects families from accepting the reality of the worst news. An honest and sincere discussion allows family members to face reality, which means that they will be able to precede a little more rationality at this angst-ridden time in their lives, when they must make so many decisions regarding the ill-health of a loved one. Because of the social worker's good work, knowledge of grief counseling, it is possible now to proceed in a more rational manner. While families adapt to the new reality, they calm themselves down, and at the same time they express more of their feelings, feelings that have perhaps been submerged for years.

For some family members this is the first time they have allowed themselves to think and talk about the reality of the situation. This is also the time when the family members can begin to make medical decisions. However, the main purpose of the meeting with the family of the patient is to ensure that the medical wishes of the patient are respected. This is the time when the family actually might even be made aware of the patient's wishes for the very first time. After all, grandma may have kept her wishes a secret until the end. Family members may have assumed that grandmother did not understand, but it turns out that grandmother understood everything. She clearly does not want to be resuscitated if and when there is an event construed as a medical emergency.

It is imperative that the family is informed and thus become aware of the patient's wishes. These wishes should not be overruled. At the same time, it is important for families to know that everything is being done to help the patient recover.

What needs to be known is the medical and psychosocial domains are forever interconnected. There cannot be a break between medical and psychosocial and yet there often is a break. The medical model is iron clad and often invites no other players. However, social work can be the basis for creating a new partnership with patients, families, physicians, and nurses, but especially when the social worker is located in the ICU, where so many tense emotions tend to be expressed.

Only the social worker has the skill-set to solve the problems that arise in a medical emergency. The social worker sets realistic goal. However, the social worker is not just being practical. This is a misunderstanding. To say that the social worker in the ICU is simply offering practical advice is once again another way to undermine the hard learned skilled of the experienced social worker. What the social worker offers, once again is a set of realistic goals that can be attained by the family in a medical crisis. In the midst of such a crisis as it unravels in the ICU, one will find the social worker doing his/her job, which is to communicate effectively with family members.

The social worker is able at this time to process a number of ambiguous messages and emotional responses that would otherwise be described as confusing. The social worker makes use of a tool belt of tools that are not just handed to him, but had to be earned, through training and through experience in the field. Even though at this time, families sometimes turn on the social worker and blame the social worker, the social worker is able to field questions, suggest alternatives, sift through the difficult decisions, and therefore in the end mobilize a number of resources that prop up the family, support the family, and ultimately work to heal the family. The family in crisis in the ICU ends up with a number of solutions that will all work to solve the problems at hand, related to the crisis, related to the sick patient, to possibly the dying patient, as well as related to the other family members as well.

Difficult Questions that Families Members Ask

1. Is my loved one going to get better?
2. Why is this happening to us?
3. How much time does my loved one have?
4. What is going to happen after he/ she passes away?

Emotional Reactions:

1. Anger; is frequently directed to others.
2. Guilt; to think that the illness or death is a "punishment" for not taking care of the patient.
3. Blame; the thought that the situation is other people's fault.

According to Kübler-Ross (1969) in her book "On Death and Dying, " people go through five stages during the lost of a family member caused by death.

1. **Commotion and Denial;** is the initial reaction when people are told bad news. They could not believe that the prognosis was true. Denial can function as a buffer after the unexpected news; it allows people to collect themselves and mobilize other defenses.

2. **Anger;** denial gives way to feelings of rage, resentment, and envy. People ask themselves the question: "Why me?" Anger can be displaced or projected toward the people around them.
3. **Bargaining;** people may bargain with God asking for more time.
4. **Depression;** anger and rage are replaced by feelings of depression. It is a phase of anticipatory grief that one may experience in order to prepare for one's death.
5. **Acceptance;** if people had enough time to go through the above phases, then they can accept the lost of their loved one. Anger, depression, and loss are no longer powerful feelings to combat; they become distant to the focus of dying.

What is new to understanding grief, it may be that it are the families that need more help than the patient at this time, more support, and understanding. This sound harsh, but it is true. The sick and suffering patient, in reality, has entered a netherworld, where the suffering has become intense. People who are not suffering do not realize the uproar around them; they are busy suffering.

When dealing with the above mentioned set of intense emotions, the social worker should seek the etiology of these emotions. Why is everyone so angry? Did the patient, when well, do something to inspire such ire? Sometimes at the bedside of a dying patient, the issue is money. This is especially sad to see, but the social worker on myriad occasions sees that the issue at hand is money. Family members are dividing up the estate of the mother, or the grandfather. They want their "fair share" of the pie. What is especially sad is when the patient knows that money is the issue. The social worker at this time is especially solicitous towards the patient, showing him/her that not everything is about money. At the same time, the social worker leads the family towards an understanding that their anger, resentment can sometimes be a displacement. The intensity comes from not being able to accept the imminent death of a loved one, or even the imminent death of a hated one.

Post-traumatic stress, anxiety, and depression are common conditions of families of patients in the ICU, especially when they have to make decisions about medical treatment, including end of life decisions about a loved one. Family members in today's hospital, in spite of all efforts to communicate more effectively, often fail the test to provide basic information about the diagnosis, prognosis, or critical care of patients. Thus, families experience tremendous levels of anxiety, frustration, and depression. As reported in the *New England Journal of Medicine,* Darmon, B., & Colleagues (2007), quantified the effects of interventions that were designed to improve the communication between the medical personnel of the ICU and family members of patients. The results of the study demonstrated that scheduled meetings with families, that offer a precise agenda, allow family members an opportunity to express their emotions and therefore in the end to make better decisions regarding the care of their loved one.

The rationale for guidance of the social worker's intervention, which helps to help families in the ICU, is based on the following:

1. To valued and appreciate what families have to say.

2. Recognize family member's emotions by doing a summary of reflective information.
3. Pay attention to what families have to say about their feelings.
4. Understand who the patient was as a person when asking straight forward questions.
5. Motivate families to ask questions.

In order for social workers in the ICU to function more intelligently, they must receive training. This training prepares social workers to intervene in ways that prepares families for bad news and good news, as well as prepares the patient for whatever lies ahead. At all the times, the social worker works on the premise that everyone has dignity, both the patient and the family. At all times, the social worker proceeds with this value (dignity, etc) planted firmly in any and all actions, as values like dignity, respect, and compassions are the hallmarks of social work practice, but especially intervention practice in the ICU of the hospital. The golden rule is an apt principle at this point, for the social worker asks the family: how would you like to be treated at this point in your life?

Family members have a consequential effect on the recovery of the patient. The families' values, beliefs, attitudes and behaviors figure prominently in whether grandmother or mother or daughter will recover speedily. Old wounds and old tensions between family members do not help the situation. However, even the most toxic family dynamics can be improved by the social worker's intervention skills, for the social worker takes care of the patient and the family at the same time. The anxiety of the patient and the family is decreased. All of this reduction in stress and anxiety equals a proportionate increase in recovery patient and family.

Intervention by the social worker has far reaching effects on the entire system, on the hospital and all hospital personnel, on doctors, nurses, and administrators. In the end, the on-going ligneous proclivities of the present society in which we live are also lessoned, for now there is more harmony, more communication, more understanding between all parties concerned. Further longitudinal studies on social work intervention in the ICU would reveal less threat of law suits. All indications so far point to this conclusion.

As the patient grows worse, sicker, the entire family structure often undergoes a transformation. The social worker has to be cognizant of these transformations. Sometimes, the patient was the matriarch or the patriarch or the power-house within the family, and now that the person is sick, or even dying, the family experiences a certain degree of confusion, even disintegration. It is not uncommon in this situation for a family member to also become ill. Grandmother might be dying of cancer, and now her adult son has a stroke or a heart attack and dies before his mother. This is not an unusual story. Stress takes its heavy toll on the human body. A son who has unresolved issues with his mother cannot tolerate his mother being terminally ill. To deal with, he himself experiences a serious medical effect, as in ischemic stroke event. Let us remember that the family is a system with its own homeostasis. To maintain balance, a family member can get sick as the previous patient actually recovers.

What Are the Needs of Families?

Based on the author's experience and observation in the ICU, patient's families have several needs. According to Freichels, T. A., (1991), these needs are grouped in five areas that are universally experienced by most families when a loved one is admitted to the ICU:

1. To feel secure; reflecting the need to keep hope and talk about the recovery of the patient. By fulfilling this need, the social workers promotes trust, sense of security and creates a doubt free environment

2. To stay near the patient; reflecting the desire of the family to stay intact, together. By fulfilling this need this gives emotional support to the patient.

3. To receive information; reflecting the understanding of the patients medical condition. By reaching this need helps the family to come to terms and make decisions and help the patient. Family's anxiety is reduced and promotes a sense of control.

4. Be comfortable; reflecting the need to reduce stress. When people are comfortable, they conserve energy and that way reduce stress.

5. Have available emotional support; reflecting in the need for expert professional help. Reaching this need helps to deal with anxiety, improves family's resources and keeps strength to help the patient.

Social Work Intervention with Families of Patients who Lack Decision Capacity

The social worker confronts many ethical situations in the ICU. One of these situations has to do with the patients' lack of decision capacity due to their critical medical condition (NASW, Code of Ethics, 2000).

Any person 18 years of age or older who is admitted to the hospital is presumed to have decision capacity to make medical decisions, unless it is indicated otherwise. Decision capacity consists in a person's ability to receive and/or to reject medical treatment. Some people cannot make medical decisions due to their medical condition or a cognitive deficiency. Lack of decision capacity is subject to various changes. For example, when a person has suffered slight a head trauma, the question is: when will he/she be able to resume his/her decision capacity? For example, if a person has suffered minor cerebral trauma, does this mean he/she can resume his/her decision capacity? What about a person who has either suffered mental retardation or is born with mental deficiency? The family has to understand that a person with mental retardation will never be able to resume his /her decision capacity. People who lack decision capacity need help from other people. However, let us be warned: some decisions can be difficult and can create ethical and professional dilemmas.

According to the NASW (2000), when a patient lacks decision capacity for medical treatment, the social worker must advocate for the protection of his/ her rights. Yet, there are dozens of instances and dozens of mitigating factors. Generally, for patients who lack decision capacity, the social worker collaborates with the medical team, and collaborates with the family, to make informed decisions about the decision making capacity of the patient. At all times, the social worker is looking for perimeters that spell out clear boundaries that are clear, as to how much diminishment of capacity has occurred in the case of the patient.

The wishes of the patient must be respected. Yet, in the end when the patient has become totally "unaware", the question always arises as to how many of the wishes of the dying patient will be respected. There are always limitations in this regard. For example, if a patient is in need and the family is very poor, can they proceed with expensive funeral plans? Is this realistic? Would it not be better to have grandmother cremated? Yet, the family could "cry out" at this defies the religious practices of the grandmother. Thus, the social worker is aware that all of these instances are not simple. Sometimes the patient is not terminal, and therefore it is a question of recovery

Once again, the values and beliefs of the patient should be respected, but there are boundaries on respect as well. Respect cannot exceed the material needs of a family. In other words, social workers cannot inflict their highest ideals on a family that cannot afford to embrace these high ideas. The best plan to follow is to have meetings with the family to figure out the needs of the family, and to proceed from this point forward. The exchange of information is invaluable. Keeping the channels of communication open is critical. The good social worker provides the family with as many good options that are possible.

The following illustration is an example of the degree of complexity of ethical decisions that face patients and family members in the ICU. The name of the patient has been altered to protect the patient's identity.

Illustration:

Mr. G. is an 85 year old man resident of a nursing home facility. Mr. G. was admitted to the hospital with severe respiratory problems and stroke. He suffered from dementia. Mr. G. did not have a Health Care Proxy. First, he was taken care in the emergency room and later he was transferred to the Intensive Care Unit (ICU). While in the ICU, the social worker was able to contact his daughter with whom a meeting was scheduled. The medical team arranged to attend this appointment as well. The attending physician explained to Mr. G's daughter that the treatment for her father was not working. Mr. G. was not responding well. The medical team spent considerable time explaining to Mr. G's daughter that the prognosis for her father was very poor. His recovery was anticipated. Other family members were also at this meeting to receive this sad news about Mr. G. The Social Worker played an instrumental role in the meeting regarding Mr. G., for it was the Social Worker who facilitated communication between Mr. G's daughter, and the rest of the family, and the Medical team. All misunderstandings about Mr. G's true condition at this time were resolved, so that when the meeting ended all family members felt satisfied that the medical team had done everything possible to restore their father and relative to health. Without the intervention of the Social Worker, family members could have gone away feeling ignored and frustrated, as the condition of Mr. G. had not in the past been properly explained. There was anger and resentments in the meeting that dissolved as the Social Worker practiced a skill-set that only belonged to him. The skills practiced here had nothing to do with the Social

Worker's compassion or intuitive powers. The skills practiced had to do with excellent training (education) and experience,

What is learned from the above example is: when a patient lacks decision capacity and is admitted to the hospital, the first job of the social worker is to find his/her family and determine if the patient has ever mentioned his/her medical wishes in the event that he/she is not able to make decisions. In the case of Mr. G, the social worker helped his daughter and other family members to identify and clarify his wishes, with the purpose of honoring (fulfilling) his wishes. The purpose of the meeting with Mr. G's family was to discuss and exchange information, and to therefore clear up any misunderstandings about the information that had been given to them by the medical team. Once again, let us notice that this was a time for questions and let us also notice that the family's intense emotions had been subdued, as answers were forthcoming from the social worker and from the medical team. Everyone present was present to resolve, decide, and determine how to proceed in the case of Mr. G who had lost his reasoning capacities through dementia.

The following family members or substitutes can give consent for medical treatment in the event that a patient lacks decision capacity:

1. - Wife (legally married).
2. - Parents.
3. - Siblings.
4. - Adult children.
5. - Adult family members.

These people are actively related to the patient.

The role of the social worker is to acknowledge and respect all parties. The social worker is used to dealing with more than one system, or one individual. There is the medical establishment; there is the social work profession; there are families; there is always a patient. All of these systems often come into conflict, and so the social worker intervenes to resolve conflicts. The social worker is trained in conflict resolution. At the same time, the social worker is acutely aware of ethical issues that pertain to the treatment of people with dementia.

Even though the above description of the social worker is apt, it turns out to be an ideal picture. On many occasions, because the hospital, the ICU, the medical staff are not prepared to cooperate, at the end of life there is often confusion, hurt feelings, terrible resentments, and bitter feelings. This is totally unnecessary. When there is a plan for care in the case of dementia cases, the outcome is very different.

The skilled social worker with experience in the ICU understands that he/she practices a set of skills that cannot be duplicated by any other person in the hospital. The doctor, nurse or family member can step up to the plate and do the job of the social worker. It is the social worker who controls communication dynamics between medical staff and family members. It is the social worker who alleviates fear, for the patient and individual family members. It is the social worker who marshals the energy of the family, to direct their collective will's towards making the end-life of their loved one comfortable, peaceful, free of worry and tension. Finally, it is the social worker who lays out the goals of the family and helps them to agree on a plan of action that meets the needs of everyone concerned: patient, medical team, family members, and the social worker.

The Social Worker as Facilitator during the Meeting with Family Members

The social worker gathers information and recommendations given by the medical team in the ICU as well as the emotional needs of family members, and their cognitive process in order to provide a sense of control, connection and meaning. Within this context the patient receives adequate medical attention while the family members are willing to learn coping skills and control their sorrows and fears of the inevitably lost of their loved one. Finally, the information and process experienced by family members during the meeting can be used to make adjustments about medical wishes as the patient's medical condition changes. The social worker can also provide support and keep the communication with families and the medical team.

Cultural Competence

There is a need for a closed communication with patients' family members. Language obstacles can be overcome when the social worker intervenes with families that do not speak English. Obstacles for a good communication, differences in attitudes about medical treatment, and other misunderstandings interfere with good medical treatment for these families. Such obstacles can be overcome when the social worker and the medical personnel are cultural competent and can guarantee good communication with patients and their families.

Lum, D. (1999) defined cultural competence as the *"group of knowledge and skills that social workers and health care professionals have in order to be competent with multicultural patients."* Multicultural social work deals with different components of culture which includes, gender, race, age, sexual orientation, religion, etc. Green, J. (1982-1999), author of "Cultural awareness in the Human Services" was right when he said that the practice of ethnical competency requires having a knowledge base, professional training, and adequate interventions in order to be able to compare and understand different cultures. As it was mentioned by Betancourt, J. R. (2004), culture is a group of learned beliefs, shared values, stiles of communication, practice, costumes, and points of view in regards to roles and relationships.

The daily activities of the author with Spanish speaking patients and their families provide an understanding about the complexity of bilingual and bicultural communication in the hospital system, especially in the ICU. These experiences can also be extended to other patients and families of foreign language. Those social workers who do not speak Spanish frequently find themselves experiencing communication problems with patients and families who do not speak English. Having had the experience of being admitted to the hospital when he first arrived to the USA and not having English proficiency and having being interviewed by medical personnel who did not speak Spanish, the author is aware of the problems that patients and their families encounter when they are interviewed by non Spanish speaking people.

Not everybody who speaks Spanish is the same. They all have different social cultural histories. The Spanish speaking countries are geographically different, have specific costumes, and have ethnic and racial mixtures. Latin-American people are associated with nineteen Spanish speaking countries in the Caribbean, Central and South America. The following countries are: Cuba, Dominican Republic, Puerto Rico, Costa Rica, El Salvador, Nicaragua, Panamá, Guatemala, Honduras, México, Bolivia, Paraguay, Uruguay, Ecuador, Venezuela, Colombia, Chile, Perú and Argentina. These countries share history and colonization, similarities in their relationship and adaptation with the Catholic Church, in their control of the Spanish language, and in their ethnic and cultural mixtures. As a result of the above mentioned, they also share cultural patterns. Cultural attitudes and beliefs are learned and better understood through conversation. To depend of translators when interviewing patients or families can be frustrating for both, patient, families and social worker. The communication is not precise and clear, even if the translator is excellent. Another frustrating factor is that social workers do not have control of the interview when they relied on the translator to interview patients, and it is difficult to obtain adequate information. An explanation for this is that the social worker can communicate directly with neither the patient nor families.

An adequate intervention with patients and families who only speak Spanish requires a strong understanding of both languages, also requires the skills to communicate efficiently in either language at different levels. Patients and family members are not trained and also they do not have the experience and can suffer a dramatic disappointment when confronted with the stress inherited in the context of the illness and hospital admission.

Social workers who intervene with non English speaking patients and family members could face challenges when evaluating their psychosocial needs, these challenges include:

1. Inadequate communication.
2. Inadequate delivery of services.
3. Inadequate definition of problems and needs.
4. Lack of understanding of the individual's functioning and family dynamics.

Problems in evaluating situations of patients and family's needs could happen when there is a lack of understanding of ethnic, cultural, social and economic contents which are important for the understanding of attitudes about the social needs and behavior. Difficulty in making assessments can also occur when the social worker does not have appropriate training for interventions in the ICU.

Conclusion:

Meetings with family members has shown to be an effective way for the members to be able to discuss emotional topics and make difficult health care decisions. Clearly the most tense is the decision to discontinue unnecessary treatments and procedures for their loved ones. By allowing family members in an open and honest space where there is enough time for them to share their emotions and discuss difficult topics, the connections among the expressed wishes and recommendations of the medical personnel can create a trusting environment. Meetings with family members help them because the shared information by the social worker is heard by all at the same time. Family members value this opportunity so they can ask questions to the social worker. This is also an opportunity to express their feelings (sorrow, sadness, cry, anger), and to show emotional support by *"touching"* and with verbal expressions of affect expressions in a quite environment.

For some family members this could have been the first time that they have allowed themselves to think and talk about the reality of the situation. If the patient was of higher family hierarchy, the meeting with the family could start the process with a new alignment and structural power. This is the moment where family conflict can start with regards to decision makings. For the majority of family members, the wish to do what is best for the patient thinking about his/her wishes helps as a motivation for working together.

The main objective of the meeting with patients' family members is to assure that patient' wishes are respected, that the family members are aware of those wishes, that they recognize that everything that needs to be done for the patient is done, and that the doctors are doing the best they can for the recovery of the patient. The social worker can clearly explain the reason and expected results at the beginning of the meeting. For example, the social worker can say; *"here we are gathering today to understand the values and wishes of your loved one, discuss his/her medical condition, what is happening with her/him now, the implications of the condition (especially prognosis for recovery), and together make possible the patient's decisions in regards to the steps to follow based on the doctors recommendations."*

The medical and psychosocial domain is connected to the health care system. The psychosocial field of social work is the basis for the creation a new relationship with patients, families, doctors and nurses in a tensed and full of emotions environment such as the ICU. The challenge for social workers is to be able to demonstrate the relevance of their intellectual capacity and clinical skills and to be able to understand the different emotional needs of family members. Control of psychosocial, spirituals practices of families are the basis for an efficient intervention to solve problems.

The practical aspects of establishing realistic goals of medical attention among health care professionals, communicating in an efficient way with families therapeutically, and helping to make sense in the experience are important for the family. Meetings with family members in the ICU is important because it is an excellent tool to create an environment of honest communication focusing in mobilizing the available resources for the patient, the family and the medical personnel towards a common plan of action.

REFERENCES

Aguilera, D. & Messick J K (1974). Crisis intervention: Theory and Methodology. St. Luis: C.V. Mosby Co. p. 631

Betancourt, J. R. (2001). Cultural Competence—Marginal or Mainstream Movement? New England Journal of Medicine; 351-953-955

Curtis, J. R, Patrick D L, Shannon S E. (2001). The Family conference as a focus to improve communication about end of life care in the Intensive Care Unit. (suppt): N 23-26

Darmon, B., Lautrette, A, Megarbane, L. M., Chevret, C Bleichne, C., Bruel, G., Choukroum., (2007). A Communication Strategy and Brouchure for relatives of Patients Dying in the ICU. New England. L. Med., 356 (5): 469-478.

C, Adrie, A., Barnaut, G, Bleichner, C. Bruel, G., Choukroun et al. (2007). Bleichner. C., Bruel G., Choukroum et al. (2007). A Communication Strategy and Brouchure for Relatives of Patients Dying in the ICU. New England. L. Med., 356(5): 469-478

Department of Medicine (2007). Bronx Lebanon Hospital Center. Bronx New York.

Freichels T A. (1991). Needs of family members of patients in the Intensive Care Unit over time. Crit. Care Nurs. Q. 14(3):16-29

Green, J. (1999). Cultural Awareness in the Human Services 2nd ed. Englewood Cliffs, NJ: Prince Hall.

Green, J. (1999). Cultural Awareness in the Human Services 3rd ed. Englewood Cliffs, NJ: Prentice Hall.

Kira, P; Kira I Kristtjanson (2004). What do patients receiving Palliative care for cancer and their families want to be told. An Australian and Canadian Qualitative Study. B M. J; 328-1343

Kübler-Ross E. (1969). On Death and Dying: What the dying has to teach Doctors, Nurses, Clergy, and their families. Publisher: Simon & Scuster Adult Publishing Group Number1

Lum, D.(1999). Cultural Competence Practice. Pacific Grove, CA: Books/Cole.

National Association of Social Workers (2000). Code of Ethics of the National Association of Social Workers. Washington DC: Author.

CHAPTER FOUR

Social Work Intervention with Families of Patients With Dementia in the Intensive Care Unit

What is Dementia?

ACCORDING TO THE ALZHEIMER'S Association (2010), the term dementia is used to describe a group of symptoms, which include a serious deficit in the memory (abnormal changes in the brain), and difficulties in one of the following areas:

1. Social functioning (confusion with time, place), affecting the functioning at home/social events and work site.
2. Changes in personality (confusion, careless in appearance).
3. Difficulty to think (difficulty to plan or solve problems and complete assignments such as: pay bills).
4. Deterioration of judgment.

Dementia is the most common form of Alzheimer's disease. This illness takes the name of Alois Alzheimer who in 1906 examined the brain of a 51 year old woman after she died who was apparently suffering from Dementia (Veterans Administration Medical Center, 1989).

There are 70 causes of dementia; Alzheimer's disease is the most common and includes between 50%-75% of old dementias. According to a report from the Alzheimer's Association (2010): "Regarding the facts and numbers of the Alzheimer's disease, there are as many as 5. 3 million people in the United States alive with Alzheimer's disease." Alzheimer's and other dementias triple the cost of health care in Americans 65 year old or older; and every 70 seconds somebody develops Alzheimer's disease (Alzheimer's Association, 2010). According to the same report, Afro-Americans and Latinos have a higher probability to develop Alzheimer's, but less probability of being diagnosed early." Alzheimer's shows abnormalities in the brain, commonly referred to as plates and balls. The size of the brain diminishes significantly and the plates and balls affect the parts of the brain that control: speech, how to solve problems, handle emotions, reactions to sensory stimulation, special navigation and judgment. Every day people with dementia are less able to take care for themselves. Dementia does not distinguish between race and cultures and the experience is similar in all ethnic groups (Alzheimer's Association, 2010).

Any person 18 years old or older who is admitted to the hospital, unless it is otherwise indicated has decision capacity, which is determined by the patient's ability to receive or reject medical treatment. Some people cannot make decisions due to his/her medical condition or cognitive deficiency. Lack of decision capacity is subject to various changes. For example, a person who has suffered a small injury to the brain can resume his/her decision capacity. People with mild and even relatively severe concussions recover fully all the time. However, a person with dementia has lost complete capacity to make meaningful decisions that reflect the best interest of the one presumably making those decisions.

A person with dementia needs help from other people. However, the social worker must be on the lookout, for certain decisions that create real ethical dilemmas, wherein the decisions made by all, everyone of them, produce difficult dilemmas. For example, sometimes the social worker is forced to advocate for the cessation of medical treatment without actually knowing the precise wishes of the patient. The social worker walks away from this scene feeling frustrated, confused, even angry, for all the good advice given about the patient's deteriorating condition was left unheeded. Thus, sometimes it is the social worker who has to work through certain unresolved issues about patients and families going their own way and not listening to expert professional advice that comes hard earned, from tough training and lived experience in the field.

According to the National association of Social Workers (NASW, 2002), when a patient does not have decision capacity for his/her medical treatment, and there is not documentation about his/her medical decisions (Advance Directives), it is confusing to say who actually represents the patient, or who will be advocating for the patient, for the patient's interests. When this is the case, it is imperative for the social worker to keep in close contact with the medical team and the family of the patient.

For patients with dementia who are admitted to the ICU, the social worker advocates and collaborates first with the medical team, but then keeps the family informed at all times about the progress of the patient. It is important that the social worker communicates to the family that he/she intends to be consistent in defending the patient's final wishes (before loss of cognition) as well as consistent with the family too. There are values and beliefs that must be adhered to, and the social worker is the one who is acutely aware of this imperative.

Adherence to the values and beliefs of the patient, as well as the family is the reason the social worker schedules frequent meetings with family, medical team, and all concerned. The purpose of the meetings is to illuminate always what the patient would want in this case, and what would be the best course of action considering the challenging circumstances. Medical treatment has its limitations and the social worker while not afraid to discuss these limitations always wants to proceed with caution, so as not to offend the sensibilities of the family, who feel frightened and confused during these very difficult days when their loved one is now present in the ICU.

What Needs Do Families' Have—Who Have Relatives with Dementia in the Intensive Care Unit?

The ICU is the one place in every hospital where families' of patients with Dementia can expect to experience the most impact from intense emotions that can be either handled well by the social worker or handled poorly. Here in the ICU family members are exposed to the worst possible conditions: lack of privacy, annoying monitors and beeps and buzzer sounds, all kinds of extraneous noise, along with the sudden call for urgent medical procedures to be performed. Let us also remember that the ICU ends up being the place where family members will be witnesses, not only to the death of loved ones, but also the death of complete strangers in the cubicle next door.

The families' can be grouped into five categories. These five categories form an interesting typology of "family needs" that are universally experienced by family members who spend any time in the ICU (Freichkes, T. A., 1991). Families need to:

1. **Receive Security**: reflects the need to maintain hope and talk about recovery of the patient. Achieving this need promotes trust, security, and freedom from doubt.

2. **Stay near the patient:** reflects a desire to unite and maintain the relationship. This can give emotional support to the family.

3. **Receive information;** reflecting the understanding of the patient's condition.

4. **Being comfortable;** reflecting the need to reduce stress. Achieving this need can help to cope with anxiety and stress. Being comfortable helps control anxiety and stress.

5. **Having available support;** reflecting the need for expert help or assistance. Achieving this need can help cope with anxiety, improve the available resources for the family and protect the family.

Public's Understanding/Response from Governments (Administrations & Officials) about Dementia.

People around the world, as they become more aware of Alzheimer's Disease, they demand more answers from their governments to find ways to prevent and to cure this frightful disease, wherein people lose their total memory, both their short term memory and their long term memory. They are alive without a memory of who they are: without explicit memory or implicit memory.

These same people in the world are also demanding that affected families find more answers to their questions as well. According to the Alzheimer's Association's report (2010), investigations into Alzheimer's disease yielded the following result at the Alzheimer's Congress held in Washington D.C. in 2000, where 5000 people participated from nations around the world. At the conference, the audience members listened to reports broadcast on television, reviewed articles that were published in magazines, and newspapers, but all focused on the subject of Alzheimer's disease. People at this well attended conference also listened to ideas about alternate treatment possibilities.

The outcome of the conference was significant, for now the disease of Alzheimer's had been placed on the international map; it had gained in status. However, in spite of the numerous medical interventions analyzed, categorized, and typologies, not a single speaker spoke on the subject of the Alzheimer patient in the ICU. Yet, most Alzheimer's patients end up in the ICU. This indicates that what many people at the conference perhaps did not and still do not realize is: the end action of Alzheimer's Disease takes place in the hospital in the Intensive Care Unit, with family members, the patient, the medical team, and the lone social worker, who tries to invent communication conduits as he/she goes about the arduous task of directing the final days of the Alzheimer's Patient. Even if the social worker at this point flounders, it does not matter. He/she has no book to follow or manual to read for a guide, and thus it might be this document presently being read that might be the first single one that speaks so specifically to the problems encountered by the social worker in the ICU, as he/she attempts to attend to the Alzheimer's patient, the patients' family, and the medical team.

Social Work Intervention with Families of Patients with Dementia in the Intensive Care Unit

The Intensive Care Unit (ICU) is the place in the hospital where attention is given to patients in the midst of a critical care crisis (life threatening). This means that one or more vital organs have been compromised, and other vital organs are soon to follow. At this point in time, exacting intervention is required by the medical team, but also required by the social worker, who goes to work immediately trying to ascertain the situation, which means see the patient, establish contact (as much as possible), while at same time establishing contact with family members, and the often obdurate medical team, who sometimes insist on following protocols that are blatantly absurd to follow when the patient has advanced stages of Alzheimer's Disease.

In the midst of this chaos where we find the Alzheimer's patients in the ICU, the social worker has a clear role to play in the life of the patient, as well as the lives of the family members. His/her intervention skills will be keenly appreciated at this point. First, the social worker labors to protect the legal rights of the patient who has lost awareness of him/herself.

Second, the social worker, once again, schedules meetings that will keep the channels of communication open between family members and the rest of the medical staff, the doctor and nurse, as well as any other health care professionals. Let us remember that it is the social worker who is trained in the dynamics of family interactions. It is the social worker who will know what the family wants and what the family means, whether the family expresses things explicitly or implicitly.

Once again, because of certain, precise skill-set the social worker in the group will be the one who knows about the "group" and knows about the intense emotions that are being thrown back and forth between family members, distraught over the condition of their loved one with dementia. The social worker has the ability to field questions and even ask pointed questions, to attain a level of awareness of the situation, to bring everyone in the ICU to a better understanding of the patient and the true nature of dementia, and or Alzheimer's disease. For it is the social worker who understands the disease as an obsessive thief who cannot stop robbing the patient of his mind, his memories, his life.

The social worker needs to have interpersonal and professional skills to allow him/her relate with people in especial conditions, different from those that are found in other professional fields. At the same time should incorporate knowledge that supersedes his/her discipline (Novoa, M., & Ballesteros, D. E., 2006). Time and duration of the meeting with family members varies due to the number of members present, the complexity of situation, and the needed time to express feelings, the need to gather additional information from the medical team, and the ability to reach an agreement between the families and the medical team. The social worker could be able to identified conflicts within the family members which could be utilized against an agreed decision. Keeping the focus of attention in what could be best for the patient can help to overcome problems, differences and conflicts among family members.

Although many of the resources and guidelines of communication are available, one of the most practical ways to facilitate communication about its context has been described by Kira, P. & Kira, j., (2004), which included:

1. To be fair,
2. maintain course of action,
3. give time,
4. show that people are important,
5. cover all important information.

Actually there are not formulas that meet the needs of families of patients admitted to the ICU.

The social worker in the ICU organizes the information and recommendations given by the medical team with the emotional needs of family members in their cognitive process in order to increase the sense of control, connection and meaning. Within this context the patients receive the best medical care, while their families are more willing to learn coping skills in order to control their fears of a possible loss of a loved one. Finally, the information and process experienced by the family members during the meeting with the social worker can be utilized to make decisions base on the patient's wishes. The social worker provides emotional support by keeping open communication with family members and the medical team.

During the patient's admission to the ICU, communication with family members is an important component of social work practice. Family members are given the opportunity to ask questions, express their feelings and fears.

The following is an example that has to do with ethical decisions in regards to the end of life of a patient with dementia. The name has been altered to protect the identity of the patient.

Illustration:

Mr. Mario is an 80 year old man living in a Nursing Facility and has Alzheimer's. Mr. Mario was taken by ambulance to the hospital emergency room and was later admitted with heart failure. On his arrival to the ER, he did not have documented Health Care Proxy and neither advanced directives. After his admission in the ER he was transferred to the Intensive Care Unit (ICU). Once there the social worker was able to locate his daughter via telephone and she was informed of Mr. Mario's admission. A meeting to discuss his medical condition was arranged with the attending physician who explained to the daughter about his condition and how he was not responding to treatment. His condition and poor prognosis for recovery were explained to Mr. Mario's daughter and to other family members there present. The social worker intervened by promoting communication between the family and the medical team, the treatment being provided was discussed as well as medical decisions in the event of heart failure. This was the moment where emotional support provided by the social worker was important for his daughter and family members since they were in a state of shock with the information that was given to them by the medical team.

When a patient who is admitted to the hospital and does not have decision capacity to make medical decisions and having the probability of poor prognosis for recovery, and does not have documented Advanced Directives, the social worker meets with family members or friends to discuss and find out if the patient has mentioned to any of them about his medical wishes in the event that he/she is not able to do so. The social worker is an expert in finding out new and different ways for people in these circumstances have the best relationship among themselves, considering their limitations. In Mr. Mario's case, the social worker assisted his daughter and other family members to identify and clarified his medical wishes, values and beliefs. The purpose of the meeting with his daughter and other family members was to discuss and exchange information as well as to understand their understanding about the information given by the medical team and for them to make questions.

The following family members or agents of the patient can give authorization for medical treatment in the event that the patient lacks decision capacity:

1. Wife (legal).
2. Parents.
3. Siblings.

4. Adult children.
5. Adult family members.

These people are actively involved with the patient.

The social worker acknowledges and respects their opinion. The social worker works with multiple social systems and is aware of individual differences, solving conflicts that are consistent with values, ethics and norms of the social work profession. Meetings with family members can help to have an honest discussion about treatment plans.

Conclusion:

Meetings with families of patients with dementia in the ICU show to be of importance because the members have the opportunity to discuss emotional topics and at the same time make difficult decisions. Obviously the most stressful of them is to discontinue unnecessary medical treatment when the prognosis for recovery of the patient is poor. In order to be able to discuss families' wishes in a quiet place where there is enough time to share feelings and to discuss difficult topics can create an environment of trust. Meetings with families of patients are also important because the information given by the social worker is heard by all members at the same time. Family members have the opportunity to express their feelings (sorrow, fear, guilt, anger, depression, anxiety), and to give emotional support by "touching" and with verbal expressions such as, "I'm sorry."

For some family members this could be the first time that they have had the opportunity to talk about the reality of their feelings. For the most of the family members, their wish to do the best for the patient thinking about his/her wishes and what would be the best to do helps them to work towards a common end. The main objective of the meeting with family members is to make sure that the patient's wishes are respected, that the members are aware of these wishes even before the patient lost his/her memory, and that whatever needs to be done for the better of the patient to be done, and that the medical team is doing the best that they can for the recovery of the patient.

The medical and psychosocial domain is interconnected to the heath care system. The psychosocial field of social work is the basis for the creation of a new society with patients, families and the medical team in a tensed and full of emotions environment such as the ICU. The challenge for social workers is to be able to demonstrate the relevance of their intellectual capacity and skills in order to be able to take care of the emotional needs of patients' families. To be able to handle the emotional reactions of family members in the ICU is the basis for an effective intervention to solve problems. Communication with families of patients in the ICU is important because it helps them to develop a sense of orientation with their experience. Communication is also important because it is a tool that creates a trusting environment, focused in mobilizing resources for the patients, and their families towards a plan of action that results with clear goals of medical and psychosocial interventions.

REFERENCES

Alzheimer's Association (2010). Guide for Care Takers. New York City Chapter. Magazine. Volume # 34. P.1-2

Bone RC; Mcelwee NE; Eubanks DH. (1930). Analysis of Indications for Intensive Care Unit Admissions-Clinical Efficacy Project-American College of Physicians. Chest; 104: 1806-1811.

Freichels TA (1991). Needs of family members of patients in the intensive care unit over time. Crit. Care Nurs. Q. 14(3): 16-29

Kira P; Kira I. Kristjaqnson (2004). What do patients receiving palliative care for cancer and their families want to be told. An Australian and Canadian Qualitative Study. BMJ; 328-1343.

National Association of Social Workers (2002). Code of Ethics of the National Association of Social Workers. Washington, DC: Author.

Novoa M; Ballesteros de Valderrama (2006). The Role Of the Psychologist in an Intensive Care Unit. Facultad de Psicología, Pointífica Universidad Javeriana. Bogotá, Colombia.

Veterans Administration Medical Center. Bronx, New York (1989). What is Alzheimer's disease?: Author

CHAPTER FIVE

Social Work in the Intensive Care Unit: Role Theory-Crisis Theory

S EVERAL STUDIES INDICATE THAT social workers in the hospital setting experience different perceptions and expectations about their various roles in the ICU. These various roles end up conflicting with people outside of the ICU, and with other professionals. Perceptions of the "other" are distorted. Everyone has a different idea about the role of the social worker in the ICU (Carrigan, Z., H., 1974; Cowles, Ch. & Lefcowitz, M., 1975; Davidson, K., 1990). Role theory, however, attempts to explain the interaction between individuals and organizations with emphasis on describing the exact role that the social worker performs, as well as the non-social worker. More importantly, Role theory helps the "other" to accept the roles of "others."

It turns out that Role Theory is very much influenced by the expectations of what is deemed appropriate behavior, but appropriate behavior when someone occupies a certain position and is expected therefore to play a particular role. Role theory also accounts for changes in roles, and thus changes in behavior in that particular role (Thompson, C., 2001).

Key Concepts in Role Theory

In the 4th century B.C.E., the Greek philosopher, Plato said that certain kinds (types) of people should be allowed to perform certain kinds of roles, because those types of people carried within their souls certain kinds of emotions that match their very souls. In one of Shakespeare's comedies, *"The Way You like It"*, the Elizabethan playwright wrote the famous lines . . . about roles, "All the world's a stage." It is the phrase that begins a <u>monologue</u> spoken by the melancholy Jaques in Act II Scene VII. The speech compares the world to a stage and life to a play, and catalogues the seven stages of a man's life, sometimes referred to as the seven ages of man: infant, schoolboy, lover, soldier, justice, <u>pantaloon</u>, and second childhood, "sans teeth, sans eyes, sans taste, sans everything". It is one of Shakespeare's most frequently-quoted passages. It could very well be conceived of as one of the first pronouncements about all the roles that people play in life, and all the stages they pass through before they meet their end.

Role Theory

Role theory has its sociological origins in the following authors, Cooley, Ch. H. (1902-1909) Mead, G. H. (1934); and Weber, M. (1947). However, there were others who mapped out something akin to modern role theory, a theory that persists in the fields of Psychology and Psychiatry. The "concept of role" has come to mean that someone in a role interacts within a certain system in a particular way. This suggests, however, that that same role would not be acted out in the same way in another system, which means that roles change. No one plays the same role with every single person in the same way.

Roles and the roles people play help people to bond with each other, and interact with each other in specific ways. The larger social system is composed of people playing many different roles in several contexts. People can play different roles in different contexts, simultaneously (Campton, B. R., & Galaway, B., 1989). Knowing this demonstrates that the concept of "role" is both conceptually and practically useful, but especially in social science research. The concept of "role" helps researchers to analyze the structure of social systems and to explain the behavior of the individuals within such systems (Merton, R., 1957; Davidson, K. 1990).

Merton, R. (1957), defined "role" as the demonstration of specific behavior patterns, but more than this for there are expectations that are attributed to a particular social position, and or professional/career position. Position is a particular condition in a system of relations. Position and role combine the cultural expectations of the group of relations that form social structure. The related concepts of "role" are: a) the knowledge's of the group of roles, b) and conflict of roles (Camptom, B. R & Galaway, B., 1989).

For Merton, R. (1957), people occupied "a group of roles," which is a group of identities and expectations that are socially prescribed and are associated with an acquired position. Those "groups of roles" are included in a system of social relations and different expectations. In the work environment of the author, most of the roles are performed by the Social Workers, Physicians and Nurses.

The group of roles of the social worker is acquired through socialization and professional certification (Camptom, B.

R. & Galaway, B., 1989). Education and training for the performance of a professional role is a form of secondary socialization. Primary socialization takes place during childhood and takes fundamental aspects of the person's identity, such as gender role, ethnicity, race, and social class. Secondary socialization is developed in the primary socialization and it is related with the specific formation of the group of roles that an individual occupies.

Important to the notion of complementary role and reciprocity is the fact that the role or position is combined (Camptom, B. R. & Galaway, B., 1989). If a system is going to enjoy the integration, there should be reciprocity of expectations among those who share the roles. According to Merton (1957) and Davidson (1990), the conflict of roles has two forms: **a)** Stress of position, and **b)** Stress of role. Merton, R. (1957) relates stress of position to the conflict of roles. Conflict of roles happens when there are different perceptions of what people do. In the environment of the author; doctors and nurses have a different perception of what social workers do in the hospital setting.

According to Davidson, K. (1990), the second form of role conflicts is the stress role which is a subjective experience that a person has when performing a role. There are several forms of stress role. For example; too much of a stress role is when a person thinks that his/her role is too demanding. When roles are not clearly defined, the actors experience stress because they do not know what is expected from them (Davidson, K., 1990; Oberhofer, D. B. & Simon, B. L. (1998).

According to Robins, S. P (1980); Merton, & Galaway, B. (1998), the following concepts of role theory are important for social workers:

1. -Certain roles are dictated by us and for other elements of our social system.
2. -Each role involves our own expectations, skills, and those of other people.
3. -The understanding of the role expectations implies that there are certain social norms that mark the boundaries of outside to coincide in interactions without conflicts among positions within the system and among the systems.
4. -There are certain values that are emotionally responsible in judging how people should perform their roles, from the person who occupies the position of the role and of others.

The literature shows that other professionals, specially physicians and nurses perceive the social worker as a person whose only capacity is to establish contacts with the community and provide concrete services, such as obtaining medical equipment and auxiliary services, such as arranging for transportation for patients, making telephone calls, finding clothing, public assistance, eligibility for social services, refer patients to community services (Garcés, C. M., 2002-2011).

The main role of Physicians and Nurses is taking care of patients' medical problems (diagnosis & treatment). Social work is considered an auxiliary profession which takes care of concrete services. It could be that this misconception, that limits the activities of social workers to concrete services, represent a contradiction between a legitimate, learned skill set, [that of the social worker], and the role that doctors play in the hospital and in society. Doctors have power and authority. Social workers do not have power and authority.

This present disposition of social workers, or perhaps better titled: *dis-possess-ment* as it relates to social workers in hospitals definitely slows down the smooth functioning of the hospital.

Just because social workers play numerous roles, and perform diverse tasks, does not subtract from their worth, or much needed expertise. For example we do not dismiss the advisor to the President of the United States because his title is too broad or diverse. We do not diminish the worth of advisors in any profession. If the person is advisor to the president or advisor to the CEO, or trusted advisor to any professional board, we understand that the advisor has a number of skills. We do not attempt a reduction, as we understand that a skill-set can be diverse. However, when it comes to social workers in hospitals, the medical establishment suddenly seizes with a mono-valued estimation of the social worker's worth in a place like the ICU, or Emergency or the Medical/Surgical Unit. However, this needs to change, for it is clear that social workers have established their worth in hospitals. They perform in several roles at once, with skills that draw from every discipline. This is not difficult to understand. Yet, Doctors and Nurses routinely turn Social workers into concrete "fetch" people who have big hearts and intuitive (unlearned, untrained) natures. However, the skill set of the social worker can be broken down into a very specific skill set.

An array of psychosocial problems belongs to social work. Yet, physicians and nurses perceive psychosocial problems as proper to their domain only (Cowles, L. A., & Lefcowittz, M., 1995; Cowles, L. A., 2000; Garcés, C. M., 2002). When physicians and nurses identify a patient with emotional problems, more than likely they will refer the patient to a psychiatrist who is yet another type of physician, instead of consulting with the social worker. This does not make sense, for the social worker is uniquely trained to handle the psychosocial disposition of the patient. The social worker is trained to understand and to acknowledge the impact of both environmental stress and physical stress on the patient. It is more than disappointing, therefore, for well trained social workers, who graduate from the finest social work programs in the country (Columbia University, University of Michigan, Stanford University, Yeshiva University-WWSSW), to find that their finely honed skill-set is more than under-utilized. It is misperceived as a kind of gobbled-gook that permits doctors and nurses, once again, to turn social workers into the "water boys" of the hospital. Thus, in hospitals social workers do not remain long, for they are struggling to yet play the role[s] for which they were well trained.

Social workers come to understand that the definition of their role depends on the cooperation and implied consent of other professions within the hospital setting. A word here about the author is in order, since his presence in the Bronx Lebanon Hospital has not been brief, but has expanded to include a life time, a whole career spanning twenty three years in length. Let us keep in mind that this particular hospital services some of the poorest people with the most problems of every sort in the entire country. For this reason, the doctors and nurses are generally overwhelmed. In this hospital, therefore, the skill-set of a well trained social worker has been welcomed.

There is a certain irony to this situation, that the author has been able to perform well in the various roles for which he was trained, for the doctor and nurse staff in every department, but especially in the ICU, the ER and all medical/surgical units is overwhelmed on every day of the year. There are no slow days or off days, as there would be in white, middle class suburban hospitals. Near fatal gunshot wounds, young terminal cancer patients, HIV babies, infant mortalities, multiple stabbings, wife beatings, child abuse, brutal rapes all prevail. Thus, once again, if the social worker is well trained, his/her skill set will be completely utilized, absorbed, encouraged, and developed.

With twenty three years of hospital experience behind him, the author reserves the right to speak with authority. Oddly, strangely, fortunately, all the training did not go for naught; it was used and reused, rediscovered, redistributed, and recycled.

Returning to the role of the social worker and role theory in general, now, rather than being a universally accepted role[s], it is tacked onto that part of the hospital organization that pertains to culpability, but moreover, the role of the social worker in the hospital has to do with the expectations of the organization, and how the total organization perceives the limited activities of the social worker, or the full range of activities of the social worker. Ultimately, the medical staff determines the role of the social work and how the social worker behaves with the doctors, nurses, patients and family members. Restriction of role or limitation of role depends on the doctors and nurses (Barker, R. L., 1999; Cowles, L. A., 2000; Garcés, C., 2002). It is obvious that this should not be the case.

It is wrong for other equal professionals to denigrate what roles should be played by social workers in the hospital setting. social workers in hospitals have a long standing historical presence in hospitals, going back to the turn of the 19th and 20th centuries. A short review of this long standing presence is in order here. Social work entered the hospital formally in the United States by invitation of Dr. Richard Cabot, who at the time was the Medical Chief of the Department of Medicine at the Massachusetts General Hospital in Boston, in 1905 (Davidson, K., 1990). The role of the social worker then was similar to the "Almoner" who was a person who gave free things to poor people in the form of medical attention in England.

Even though social workers have a long standing history in hospital settings, it has to be noted that there was a riff between social workers and hospital administrators from the start, for hospital administrators only wanted social workers to pin-point medical needs for doctors and nurses. More important, administrators felt that the presence of social workers would prevent hospital staff (which mainly includes doctors and nurses) from abusing the poor placed in hospitals in the first place (Davidson, K. D., Huff, D., 2008).

The continuing controversy about the real role[s] of social workers is still going strong. Nothing has been resolved; social workers in the hospital setting still attend to concrete services that take up a lot of time, but do not embrace all of the roles for which the social worker is trained: *Collaborate with other professionals to provide total care for patients; give diagnosis to psychosocial problems; be able to determine need of patients psychosocial problems; recommend psychiatric evaluations and treatment for mentally ill patients; be able to help patients to overcome crisis situations; provide emotional support; be able to use psychotherapeutic techniques; provide consultation and education to the medical personnel regarding the psychosocial problems of patients and families.*

As articulated by Davidson, K. (1990) and Cowles, L. A. (2000), social work in the hospital setting has developed into congeries *of knowledge*, which have and should have influenced the good care of the patient. Acknowledgement of the genuine psychosocial components of the social worker's skill set should be recognized as more than an auxiliary aid, and equal therefore to medical treatment.

The author here is not denying the physicality of the doctor's role, or its importance, but the author is saying that physicality is not supreme; it runs in conjunction with psychosocial components that are heart, liver, lung-like in terms of their importance. As much as *parallel tracks* is an inadequate concept, at least it speaks to the idea that one track is as important as the track on the other side. However, the idea of Tracks, suggest an antiquated linearity that should be left behind; it belongs to a previous era. The truth is: all data must be entered. in order for the patient to recover, and for the family members to thrive as well. All data is divided into datum. Once again, a systems paradigm is the optimum paradigm for understanding all hospital workers.

Social workers in the hospital setting need another *care* model for *person and family*, as the old fashioned *medical model* no longer serves any good purpose. Ultimately materiality or physicality or total emphasis on the physical has had its day. Just as the Occupational therapist works to restore FRM (Full range of motion) to the rotary cuff of the patent, so the worker in the medical profession, whether doctor, nurse, social worker (others) welcomes a model that restores full range of motion of social workers, so that they can practice all the skills in a hospital setting, for which they have been so ably trained.

To this date, there have been few studies conducted that insightfully highlight the negative perceptions of physicians and nurses, as these perceptions pertain to the role of social workers in the hospital setting (ED, MICU, Medical Surgical units). There is a need for social workers and the profession to clarify the role of the social worker in the ICU.

Social workers need to continue and to redefine and conceptualize their role within the hospital. There are always financial constraints, but these constraints do not interfere with the roles that doctors and nurses play in the hospital, and thus financial constraints should not interfere with the role that social workers play. Social workers must maintain certain values, keep congeries of knowledge's, practice a skill set, and uphold professional ethics.

Crisis Theory

During the 1950s and 1960s, psychologists of Ego Psychology, theorists like Gordon Allport, Abraham Maslow, and Eric Erikson, worked towards developing the physiological basis of crisis theory. Hippocrates, an ancient Greek physician (7th c. B.C.E.), had defined crisis: *"Crisis is a transitory or permanent event of an action or situation which puts a person's life in danger."* (Golan, N.,1978). It turns out that Crisis theory is just as important as Role Theory.

Crisis theory is defined as a group of concepts that are related, which belong to people's reactions when confronted with new experiences. These experiences could show up in natural disaster forms, illness, significant loss (family, employment), changes in social conditions, and life cycle. This theory suggests that when people experience traumatic situations, they have the tendency to follow a pattern of predictable answers (Ell, K., 1995). Crisis theory has developed because some people have short periods of anxiety and are not able to adapt to everyday problems and tensed events.

Crisis theory was developed by Linder Mann and Gerald Caplan, along with a group of sociologists, social workers, physicians and counselors. Crisis theory as a technique has its starting after the fire of the Coconut Grove in Boston, in 1994 where 493 people died in a nightclub. Crisis intervention is particularly important to social workers who find patients in the ER, MICU and Medical Surgical Units, and/or in situations of emotional traumas, despair and anxiety. Providing adequate interventions to people in severe stressed situations is part of daily practice of social workers in the hospital setting (ER, MICU, and Medical-Surgical Units). Therefore crisis intervention is of legitimate interest to social workers in hospitals.

The risk of losing a patient thru death is a present reality in the ICU. As well as the condition of the patient who is critical, there is the emotional need of families that must be considered. Family members are confronted with the shock of watching their loved one in an unfamiliar and impersonal environment, and are exposed to the suffering of neighboring patients. Sometimes, family members are asked to participate in medical decision making which in turn could exacerbate their crisis.

The social worker adjusts to the crisis and uses a variety of techniques, and thus makes a difference in the traumatic situation. The ability to make a difference to the well being of the patient and the family is the hallmark of a well trained social worker. Social work intervention in the context of crisis intervention can assist families, and help reduce the trauma that is frequently endured during the admission to the ICU. The *focus of social work is its concentration in what is going on here and now and not in the past.*

Reaction to illness and death among family members varies; some react by getting depressed, feeling guilty, anxious, scream, hold on to the medical personnel, or *walk on the halls*. Others experience panic attacks, cry incessantly, insult the medical staff, or walk away. The reaction of families of patients who are admitted to the ICU is varied, but the differences can still be typologized, categorized into patterned reactions that can be learned. The following factors need to be recognized, for these factors help the social worker to understand the varied responses to crisis and trauma.

1. Individual perception to stressful events.
2. Availability of support system.
3. Defense mechanisms to confront stressful events.

People are capable of expressing so many different feelings. The social worker's intervention is to be present, be sensitive to the emotional needs of family members, allowing family to express their feelings, provide emotional support, provide information about resources, and assure family that the loved one is receiving high quality medical care.

Dr. Elizabeth Kübler-Ross was a pioneer in developing methods of emotional support and counseling in personal trauma and depression, associated with illness and death. Her ideas enumerating the five stages of loss are useful; shock, anger, bargain, depression and acceptance. All can also be related to personal changes and emotional problems which are the result of different factors associated with death. Similar reactions can be observed in people that are confronted with different traumas such as, loss of employment, forced changes of environment, physical disabilities, victims of crime, punishment, broken interpersonal relationships, financial problems, unexpected life events, etc. (Chapman, A., 2006-2010).

Emotional stress and traumas can cause different effects in people, while death and terminal illness is for many people the last on the list of traumas. Even though it seems as if death could be handled in a different way, it turns out that people feel the same emotional discomfort when confronted with life challenges, especially if they are confronted with something difficult for the first time. If the challenges threaten weak areas, these weaknesses will manifest in different ways. Despair and anxiety (change of employment, danger, phobia, etc.) does not necessarily threaten every person. This is why it is good to understand. Crisis theory, as this model demonstrates that people's perceptions of crisis are different, from person to person.

As mentioned by Kübler-Ross (1969), people go through five stages during bereavement:

1. **Shock and despair**; it is the initial reaction of people when getting unexpected news.

2. **Anger**; could be displaced towards other people near them.
3. **Bargain**; people make deals with doctors and God in order to gain more time.
4. **Depression**; people despair and feel depressed.
5. **Acceptance**; when people had had enough time and were been able to experience the previous stages, they can accept their loss.

While the focus of attention in Kübler-Ross is death and dying, the cycle of bereavement is a useful tool to understand our emotions and of other people. Given the emphasis of crisis intervention and supportive counseling that is provided to patients and their families, it can be postulated that social work has an opportunity to make an important contribution to patient care in the hospital setting. The social worker in the hospital works with patients with chronic medical illnesses that limit their lives, cause death, and bring fears upon families, who without intervention end up in despair, anxiety and terrible stress. The traumas, psychological and psychosocial problems are real, and every patient in hospital, along with the family go through similar things; it does not matter what ethnic group they represent, or what culture; it is all the same. It does not matter what language the patient speaks, or what is the sexual orientation of the patient, or gender or what economic and social condition is in place. Trauma is the same and crisis is the same.

Social workers are constantly challenged to demonstrate their specific skill set to patients and families. At the same time they have the opportunity to influence other professional groups (physicians, nurses), and the public about their role in the hospital setting. The role social workers play is vital. The history of the social worker is a steady, unbroken chain of various accomplishments by pioneers going back to the turn of the 20th century. However, the concept of care has been around for a long time. Its history is the history of history itself, for the idea that there should be someone there to care is not new. What is new is the deconstruction of this care, into datum that can be processed into an array of data, by people who choose to work in a hospital setting. These people are Social Workers.

REFERENCES

Barker, R. L. (1999). The Social Work Dictionary, 4th ed. Washington DC: NASW Press.

Campton, B. R. & Galaway, B. (1989). Theoretical perspectives for social work practice. Social Work Process (pp. 123-141). Belmont, CA: Wadsworth.

Carrigan, Z. H. (1974). The effect of professional role on the perception of interdisciplinary social work practice in health care settings. Unpublished Doctoral Dissertation.

The Catholic University of America, Washington, DC. Chapman, A. (2006-2010). The Elizabeth Kübler-Ross: Grief Cycle. Retrieved from http:/www stages of grief.

Cooley, Ch. H. (1902). Human Nature and the Social Order, New York: Charles Scribner's Sons.

Cowles, Ch. H. (1909). Social Organization: A Study of the Larger Mind, New York: Charles Scribner's Son.

Davidson, K. (1990). Role blurring and the hospital social worker's search for domain. Health and Social Work. 15, 228-234

Garcés, C. (2002). The Social Worker in the Emergency Room. Perceptions of doctors and nurses on the role of the social worker in the emergency room. Published Doctoral Dissertation. Yeshiva University (WWSSW). New York.

Huff, D. (2008). Chapter 12. "Missionaries & Volunteers." The Social Work History Station. Boise State University. Pp. 02-20

Mead, G. H. (1934). Self and Society. Chicago: University of Chicago Press.

Merton, R. (1957). Social theory and Social Structure. New York; Free Press.

Oberhofer, D. B. & Simon, B.L. (1990). Resident guests: Social Workers in host settings. Social Work, 36, 208-211

Robbins, Stephen, P. (2008). Organizational Theory. Structure, design and implications. San Diego State University. Prentice Hall, Englewood Cliffs, New Jersey.

Thompson, C. (2001). Conservation of Theory. A Sloan Work and Family Encyclopedia Entry. Chestnut Hill, MA: Boston College.

Weber, Max (1947). The Theory of Social and Economic Organizations, ed., Talcott Parsons, Trans. AM. Henderson and Talcott Parsons. New York Press.

CHAPTER SIX

Social Work and Discharge Planning in the Hospital Setting

S OCIAL WORK AND DISCHARGE planning in the hospital setting generally implies working in collaboration with an interdisciplinary team of doctors, nurses, physical and respiratory therapists, nutritionist, utilization review case managers, as well as with other community support systems outside of the hospital (nursing homes, rehab centers, home care agencies, medical supplies agencies, etc.). In these units of the hospital the social worker prepares patients for discharge, once their medical condition has been stabilized and the patients can return to their home or to a health care facility, depending on their needs. Some patients are in need of home care services (home attendant or medical equipment, wheel chairs, walker, oxygen, etc.).

Definition of Discharge Planning

Discharge planning is an important tool for reviewing and making arrangements for on-going healthcare needs across healthcare settings, including hospitals, skilled nursing facilities, home health, or Hospice Care (Center for Medicare Advocacy, Inc. 2009). Social work and discharge planning is one facet of the larger practice of case management. Discharge planners are sometimes called "care coordinator." What exactly constitutes discharge planning is debatable and frequently depends on the setting. Broadly, the term implies linking individuals and their families with resources outside of the current setting for follow-up care (Education Resources Information Center (1999-2012).

It is the social worker's responsibility to develop a discharge plan that will meet the patient's needs and allow the patient to leave the hospital in a timely manner, so as to prevent delays in discharge that could cost thousands of dollars per day in lost revenues from third-party payers.

Admission to the hospital often brings anxiety, fear and questions to be answered for patients, their friends and families. Doctors, nurses and other care givers provide medical and technical support, but it is the social worker who provides counseling and emotional support to patients and families during what can be a stressful time. This intervention is essential to ensure a positive outcome.

The social worker is trained to work with individuals and families in dealing with personal and interpersonal crisis caused by illness and hospitalization. The social worker's role is varied and complex one, but in all cases, the social worker plays a vital part in maximizing wellness during the patient's hospital stay and in easing the transition back home or to a health care facility.

The social worker assists with teaching about advanced directives, appropriate discharge planning and counseling to patients and their families. During the patient's hospital stay, the social worker provides invaluable services that cannot be duplicated by other hospital personnel.

Example

During the medical rounds the social worker is informed that a patient will soon be "cleared for discharge" and will need home care services. It is the social worker's responsibility to arrange home care services to be in place by the date that the patient is scheduled to be discharged. If the home care service is not in place at time of discharge, the patient may not leave the hospital, resulting in a delay in discharge and the patient being placed on an alternate level of care status until the necessary services are arranged. In such situations, the treating physician is ultimately responsible for the delay.

The social worker's role is a varied and complex one, but in all cases, the social worker plays a vital part in maximizing wellness during the hospital stay and in easing the transition back home or to a health care facility. The goal of social work includes assisting patients with their advanced directives, appropriate discharge planning and counseling for patients and family members' reaction to the impact of illness and hospitalization. The social worker collaborates with other members of the interdisciplinary team who are directly involved in the patient's care.

While the patient is still admitted to the hospital,

The Social Worker:

1. Facilitates family involvement in discharge planning.
2. Keeps the family informed of the patient's progress and explains how the family can help the patient.

3. Utilizes the process of discharge planning to help the patient and the family to better understand the stress connected to illness, and the effect that this stress has on the family system as a whole.
4. Communicates with patients, families and staff.
5. Establish a therapeutic relationship with patients and family members.
6. Advocates for the patients.
7. Collaborates and coordinates discharge planning with the interdisciplinary team.

The social worker is trained to help patients and families help themselves. Assist in acquiring the tools to cope with troubling situations such as:

1. Traumatic and chronic illness.
2. Alcoholism and/or drug dependency.
3. Financial and emotional strain of caring for a disabled family member.
4. Family relationship problems due to illness/ hospitalization.
5. Elder abuse and domestic violence.
6. Bereavement/death.

Discharge planning should begin with the patient's admission to the hospital; this will allow everyone to focus on a clear endpoint in the patient's care. It also will reduce errors and unnecessary delays along the patient pathway. Review of the literature shows that there is not enough research done by social workers on discharge planning. On the other hand the literature shows that discharge planning has been studied by nursing researchers over the past several years, especially since there has been an effort to shorten length of stay for hospitalized patients (Hager, 2010).

The average length of stay for hospitalized patients has been shortened by three days for patients across all age groups and by seven days in older patients since 1970. In response to shorter length of stay, past research suggests that the profession of social work recognized early on that there were gaps between hospital and community based healthcare agencies charged with continuity of care, transfer information between providers, and discharge education of patients and families (Hager, 2010. As pointed put by Foster, J. F; Murff, Peterson, J. F; Gandhi, T & Bates, D. W. (2003), there are reports of patient's describing lack of inclusion in the discharge process, families questioning their ability to care for patients at home, a shortage of outpatient resources such as public health or home care agencies that can help patients with the transition. What went wrong with these discharges? And how did some patients return home without the information and confidence they needed for a successful transition? What is the cost of this nation's health care system and what is the cost to the patients we serve when we fail to provide adequate discharge planning to hospital patients?

Foster, Clark, Menard, Dupuis, Chernis, R & Chandok, N. (2004) suggested that nearly a quarter of medical patients experienced adverse events within one month of discharge with some preventable and some being a direct cause of treatment. One third of these events were associated with disability and one-half required additional health services. Adverse events included errors in medication orders or prescription filling, infection, confusion about discharge teaching, and failure to follow up unresolved problems.

Lack of interdisciplinary team involvement, lack of patients and families feeling included in the discharge process, and known adverse events which included patients being sent home without necessary vital equipment, without clear understanding of how to manage their care, and calls post-discharge regarding who to call with problems that had developed. At times, the lack of care coordination and adaptation of patients' medical and psychosocial needs resulted in delays in discharge. Improving patient satisfaction as well as reducing post-discharge adverse events are relevant measurements of a successful discharge process, and social workers bring a unique perspective of caring to this process, social workers assume a vital role in providing and developing and safe, cost effective, discharge planning.

Given the complexity of the discharge process, Medicare has set forth recommendations mandating a discharge plan be in place to identify patients who are likely to suffer adverse events post-discharge. It further stipulates that health care organizations provide discharge planning evaluations by licensed personnel who account for patients' capacity for self-care and availability of post-hospital services. They must show documentation of the process in the medical record, evidence of family inclusion in the process, and reassessment of the discharge plan to account for change in condition (Department of Health and Human Services, 2004). Other accrediting organizations, such as The Joint Commission on Accreditation of Healthcare Organizations (JCAHO), recommend that a discharge plan be developed that is based on appropriate levels of continuing care and exchange of patient information with other providers and health care professionals (Department of Health and Human Services, 1997).

Within the current health care system, patients are discharged from the hospital earlier as limited resources are spread over larger groups. Consideration of who will receive services will fall on the shoulders of social workers and other health providers. Taking action for social justice involves working toward reducing system-wide differences that disadvantage specific groups and prevent those groups from receiving adequate health care services. The elderly population accounts for a disproportionately high percentage of health care dollars and as our population ages, our health care system will undoubtedly be faced with decisions that may include rationing of health care services (Hager, J. S., 2010). As health care institutions search for areas to cut cost, social workers must advocate that discharge planning should not be included in budget cuts, because through discharge planning and anticipation patient needs post discharge has the potential to save the organization money through prevention, safety and patient satisfaction (Hager, J. S., 2010).

Hage, S. & Kenny, M. (2009), claim that encouraging the infusion of social and cultural diversity in health care education encounters can affect a person's worldview. Cultural issues related to disease management or health care prevention can be linked to how a particular community defines itself in the health care arena. For example, if a person of another culture refuses services because of unsubstantiated fears or beliefs, this will impact the health care providers' ability to successfully care for this patient and may result in undue harm or risk related to those e beliefs (Hager, J. S., 2010). Chadiha, L; Proctor, E; Monroe-Howel, N; Darkwa, O. & Dore, P.

(1995), found that African American patients discharged from the hospital used fewer formal services and had more tentative discharge plans due to a false assumption of increased caregiver availability than their white counterparts.

As a profession, social work can lobby for improve discharge education and planning by applying a framework of acting, and transforming on issues that negatively affect discharge planning in their organizations. First, social workers must act to alleviate symptoms of psychosocial problems, by familiarizing themselves with the issues. Secondly, social workers should reflect on the problems or issues and ask themselves, "Why are patients leaving the hospital without adequate discharge planning or education?" Listen to those affected by the problem and ask the deeper questions that challenge the current social structure; explore the underlying causes of these issues (Hager, J. S., 2010). The social work profession must develop a plan or take a different route of action in regard to the health care/psychosocial issue. Transforming action looks at the root of the problem and does not stop at alleviating symptoms. As social workers we can assist the patient that we serve with successful, seamless discharges by empowering them to become self-advocating and independent health care consumers.

Ethical Decision Making Among Hospital Social Workers

According to Kadushin, G. & Egan, M. (2001), ethical decision making represents a process of dealing with ethical dilemmas in social work. This process essentially consists of the following steps; determining if there is a conflict, whether harm has occurred; and developing a plan of action. Social workers have a duty to maintain the confidence of their clients, but if a client threatens to harm his/herself or others, the social worker also is obligated to report that. This presents a conflict between a duty to maintain confidentiality and principles as a human being to prevent harm to another person. As pointed out by Reamer, F. (1985), "Ethical decision-making is a process, and social workers should take into consideration all the values, principles, and standards in this Code that are relevant to any situation in which ethical judgment is warranted, decisions and actions should be consistent with the spirit as well as the letter of this Code." It seems that when ethical dilemmas arise, the Code's standard regarding interdisciplinary collaboration and guidelines will be a critical point of reference and may assist in clarifying for a social worker when one might be wading in "muddy" water.

Example:

During the medical rounds, the social worker is informed that a frail elderly patient, who lives alone and does not have family, is medically cleared and will be discharged with home care services. However, after assessing the patient's psychosocial needs, the social worker has determined that the patient does not have the ability to direct the home attendant and recommends that the discharge be deferred pending further assessment of the problem and the development of an alternative discharge plan that will better ensure the patient's safety. In such cases, it is the social worker's ethical duty to inform the medical team that the discharge may place the patient at risk and advocate for another, more appropriate discharge plan even if it means that the patient's discharge has to be delayed. It is in such cases as these that the social workers prove their worth by placing the needs of the patient ahead of all other considerations.

Skills Needed in Discharge Planning

1. To be able to work in collaboration with other members of the interdisciplinary team.
2. Excellent analytical skills and clinical assessment.
3. Able to communicate efficiently with the interdisciplinary medical team, patients, family members and community services.
4. To be able to establish a therapeutic relationship with patients and family members.
5. To be willing to advocate for patients' rights, especially when the social worker has identified problems that could complicate the discharge planning and put the patient in danger.

What is an Ethical Dilemma?

Kadushin, G. & Egan, M. (2001) define ethical dilemmas to those occurring when it is necessary to choose between ethics that appear contradictory. Ethical dilemmas present conflicts between social workers, other staff, agencies, clients or regulators. Social workers operate under broad ethical principles which are based on six core values: *a) service, b) social justice, c) dignity and worth of the person, d) importance of human relationships, e) integrity, and f) competence* (NASW Code of Ethics, 1999). According to

Cole, P. L. & Sparks, J. (2006), before attempting to identify, understand, and comment on ethical dilemmas, social workers should examine their personal values. Understanding differences in individual value basis has special relevance as practitioners interact with clients operating from value positions different from their own.

As pointed out by Beauchamp, T. L. & Childres, J. F. (1994), the purpose of ethics in health care is not new. Since the days of Hippocrates, medical ethics have been concerned with the ethical obligation of health care professionals in meeting the needs of the sick and injured. However, technological developments in medicine, the rapid emergence of managed care in the delivery and reimbursement of health care costs and expanding information systems have contributed to the increased frequency and complexity of bioethical dilemmas for all health care professional, including social workers. Several factors have had impact on the growing frequency of ethical dilemmas in health care.

While scientific developments in medicine have offered expanded opportunities for treatment choices and the potential for longer life, they have additionally created ethical dilemmas involving issues related to quality of life, informed consent, end-of-life decision-making including the provision for or withdrawal of life support, access to health care, and resource allocation (Blumenfield, S. & Lowe, J., 1987; Cosson, J., 1997). These developments have raised questions for social workers as to what should be done in life or death situations, who should decide, and what criteria should be used in the decision-making process (Blumenfield, S. & Lowe, J. 1987). Social work in today's environment not only requires an awareness of the clinical and ethical concerns that arise in practice, but demands a demonstration of a reasoned response toward ethical analysis and decision-making (Boland, K., 2006).

Advancements in medical technology and related ethical issues and questions affect social work practice on a daily basis. Traditionally, the function of hospital social work focused on the development of a variable post hospital plan to meet the medical and social services needs of patients (Boland, K., 2006; Blumenfield, S. & Lowe, J., 1987; Cockerman, C., 1997). These issues often present the social worker with the task of initiating ethical discussion and deliberation and demonstrating a level of ethical competence which is best approached using a reasoned process for ethical resolution (Reamer, F., 1998 & Boland, K., 2006).

Further reduction in hospital stays, less than adequate discharge plans, disposition problems and delayed discharges create many ethical conflicts for social workers' attempting to balance the competing needs of client best interest and responsibilities to the health organization, the third party payer, the medical staff and the patient's family members (Abramson, 1981; Cummings, S. & Cockerman, C., 1997 & Boland, K., 2006).

Conclusion:

Discharge planning should begin during the patient's admission to the hospital, with inclusion of the family during the process, as well as the identification of obstacles and goals of the discharge planning. This will help for the social worker to focus in the identification of patients psychosocial problems. The start of the discharge planning at the moment of the admission to the hospital will also help with cost control by preventing unnecessary readmissions and improve patient satisfaction. Ethical issues in health care continue to be a professional challenge for social workers, the process and strategies for ethical resolution need to be studied in order to understand options of resolutions that are used by social workers when trying to identify ethical situations during the discharge planning.

Frequently social workers have large case loads and have to meet tight deadlines for arranging discharge planning. Social workers in the hospital setting often deal with highly complex cases involving patients who come to the hospital with multiple psycho-social issues, all of which require assessment and treatment. Social workers treat cases involving lack of health insurance coverage, homelessness, chronic unemployment, legal problems, alcohol and drug abuse, victims of domestic violence, elderly abuse. Any of these problems can impede timely discharge from the hospital. Sometimes situations as seemingly mundane as the patient needing car fare, clothing or shoes can lead to delays in discharge, especially if these needs are not identified early upon admission to the hospital.

As ethical issues in health care continue to challenge social workers professionally, the processes and strategies for ethical resolution need to be studied and clarified in order to understand the resolution options used by social workers to address ethical issues and discharge planning. To continue the progress achieved to date, we must continue to redefine our roles within the changing, financially oriented health care environment, while simultaneously preserving our social work values, knowledge, skills, and ethics.

REFERENCES

Abramson, M. (1981). Ethical dilemmas for social workers in discharge planning. Social Work in Health Care, 6(4), 33-42.

Abramson, M. (1983). A Model for organizing an ethical analysis of the discharge planning process. Social Work in Health Care, 9(1), 45-52.

Beauchamp, T. L., & Childress, J. F. (1994). Principles of biomedical ethics (4th ed). New York: Oxford University Press.

Blumenfield, S. & Lowe, J. (1987). A template for analyzing ethical dilemmas in discharge planning. Health and Social Work, 12, (1) 47-56.

Boland, K. (2006). Ethical Decision-Making Among Hospital Social Workers. Journal of Social Work Values and Ethics, Volume 3, Number 1.

Center for Medicare Advocacy, Inc. 2009). Medicare And Discharge Planning: Think Through Your Needs.

Cossom, J. (1992). What do we know about social workers ethics? The Social Worker, 60 (3) 165-171.

Chadiha, L., Proctor, E., Morroe-Howell, N., Darkwa, O., & Dore, P. (1995). Post hospital home care for

African-American and White elderly. The Gerontologist, 35 (2), 233.

Cole, P. L. (2012). You want me to do what? Ethical practice interdisciplinary collaborations. Virginia Commonwealth University. Journal of Social Work Values and Ethics, Volume 9, Number 1.

Cummings, S. & Cockerman, C. (1997). Ethical dilemmas in discharge planning for patients with Alzheimer's disease. Health and Social Work, 22(2). 101-108.

Department of Health and Human Services. (1997, December). Medicare Hospital Discharge Planning (OEI-02-9400320). Retrieved October 2, 2010, from http://hhs.gov/ oei-02-94-00320.pdf.

Department of Health and Human Services. (2004, August). Condition of participation: Discharge Planning (42 C. F. R. 482.43). Retrieved October 21, 2010, fromhtt://law. justia.com/us/cfr/title 42/423.0.5.21.3.199.12. html.

Foster, J; Peterson, J.F., Gandhi, T. & Bates, D. W. (2003). The incidence and severity of adverse events affecting patients after discharge from the hospital. Ann Intern Med. 138(3), 161-167.

Foster, A. J., Clark, H. D., Menard, A., Dupuis, N., Chernish, R. & Chandok, N. et al. (2004). Adverse events among medical patients after discharge from hospital. Canadian Medical Association Journal, 170(3), 345-349.

Hage, S., & Kenny, M. (2009). Promoting a social justice approach to prevention: Future directions for training, practice, and research. Journal of Primary Prevention, 30, 75-87.

Hager, J. S. (2010). Effects of a Discharge Planning Intervention on Perceived Readiness for Discharge. St. Catherine University. St. Paul-Minnesota.

Kadushin, G., & Egan, M., (2001). Ethical Dilemmas in Health Care: A Social Work Perspective.

National Association of Social Workers (1996). Code of Ethics. Washington, DC: author Reamer, F. (1985). The emergence of bioethics in social work. Health and Social Work, 10, (4) 271-281.

Spehar, A., M., Campbell, R., R., Cherrie, C., Palacios, P., Scott, D., & Baker, J., et al (2001). Seamless care: Safe patient transitions from hospital to home. Advances in Patient Safety, 1, 79-97.

Sparks, J. (2006). Ethics and Social Work in Health Care. In S. Gehler & T. A. Browne (Eds.) Handbook of Health Social Work (pp.43-69). Hoboken, NJ: Wiley and Sons.